The HEADACHE HANDBOOK

Diagnosis and Treatment

The HEADACHE HANDBOOK

Diagnosis and Treatment

Gary W. Jay, M.D., D.A.A.P.M.

CRC Press
Boca Raton London New York Washington, D.C.

Library of Congress Cataloging-in-Publication Data

Jay, Gary W.
The headache handbook : diagnosis and treatment / by Gary W. Jay
p. cm.
Includes bibliographical references and index.
ISBN 1-57444-221-X (alk. paper)
1. Headache—Handbooks, manuals, etc. I. Title.
[DNLM: 1. Headache—diagnosis. 2. Headache—therapy. WL 342
J42H 1998]
RC392.J38 1998
616.8 ' 491—dc21
DNLM/DLC
for Library of Congress

98-24219
CIP

International Standard Book Number 1-57444-221-X
Library of Congress Card Number 98-24219
Printed in the United States of America 1 2 3 4 5 6 7 8 9 0
Printed on acid-free paper

Introduction

Another day, another book to read. What a pain in the neck. Or is it?

This book is about the diagnosis and treatment of headache. Its purpose is to acquaint you with just that. It goes into depth in those areas requiring such coverage but does not go *too* deeply into areas that you perhaps do not need to do your job. With an appropriate background in medicine, you can be a headache specialist, should you so choose.

The book is written, it is hoped, in a much less formal style than the typical textbook. The information should be accessible to you, the reader, so I have tried to write it in a more "talky" style, in much the same way I would present the information at a lecture.

Your job, should you choose to accept it, is to learn the information found here, if you don't already know it. It will help you if you are a general practitioner acting as a gatekeeper for an HMO or another form of managed care company, and it will help you appreciate the complexity of diagnosing and treating headache.

Why was this book written? Because a lot of people have asked me to write it, over the course of the last several years, and because I think such a source is important for physicians or clinicians of all types, generalist or specialist, to understand headache, which is possibly the most ubiquitous symptom in medicine.

On a personal note, I hate closed minds. I, like you, run into them all the time. You know, the ones who say, "I've been treating xxxxx the same way for the last decade. Why would I want to change?" or some other such nonsense. I find it difficult to deal with "authorities" who blatantly ignore facts. I have trouble talking to people who blithely state that "muscles have nothing to do with headache" and "trigger points in muscle are not real". These folk ignore years of literature and some phenomenal research, because they do not fit into their medical "world view". Or, they "weren't taught that in medical school."

I once lectured on the same podium as an extremely well-known (and deservedly so) headache specialist. The topic was the effectiveness of physical therapy on the treatment of chronic daily headache. After my talk, this expert, who was moderating the afternoon session, stated that he didn't think muscles had anything to do with headache. As nicely as I could, I reminded him that he had just published an excellent book on headache which had a chapter dealing with muscle spasm headache, or tension headache, as it was known in the mid 1980s. He wrote about it, but didn't believe it.

I don't get it.

I've spoken to clinicians who have told me, at various times, that rehabilitation, interventional anesthesiology, and especially, God forbid, manual medicine have no place in the diagnosis and treatment of headache. They even intimated that I was crazy for considering the use of such things. Well, doing what I do the way that I do it gives me exceptional results. Our outcome data indicate that over 90% of our headache patients leave treatment with no headache at all, or with headache of minimal duration and severity and vastly decreased frequency (a .5 to 2 on a visual assessment scale, with an average start at 8.5).

This book you have in your hands will tell you how I do it, what strategies I use, and why. Unfortunately, you have to understand the pathophysiology of the headache entities, how to make the correct diagnoses, the pharmacology and pharmacokinetics of medications (as in how they work, why you have to understand the physiological reasons for rehabilitation, what types to use — why, when, and for how long). Your mind has to be open enough to understand when and why to use interventional anesthesiological procedures. You have to be open enough to try manual medicine for certain problems that physical therapy cannot fix within a reasonably short amount of time.

We are all in a spot of trouble. All of us clinicians. The problem is managed care. Well, actually, managed care — while maybe not your friend — is not *really* the problem. The problem is that people, even (or especially) those who do not know the medicine but who are part of those organizations, are directing the care to those of us on the front line of medicine seeing patients. Telling us what to do and how to do it. The "whys" apparently don't matter, really.

Will this book help with this problem? Of course not. But, it may show enough clinicians who are not (yet) headache specialists the many aspects of medications, rehabilitation, and interventional procedures or manual medicine consultation. That way, there can be some form of cross-talk by people knowledgeable in the realities of diagnosing and treating headache.

Writing this book was fun for me and gave me chance to give myself a different perspective as to some of the information presented here. I hope it has a purpose and will be useful to clinicians of all types in any number of ways —like adding another specialty aspect to your practice and doing it correctly. Who wouldn't like to do that? Let's get on with it!

The author

Gary W. Jay, M.D., was practicing pain medicine even before the advent of the medical specialty, which he helped form. He did his neurology residency at Northwestern University in Chicago and has practiced pain medicine for his entire career.

He was one of the original founding members who met in Washington, D.C., in 1983 to start the American Academy of Algology, now the American Academy of Pain Medicine. He is a fellow of that organization and also board certified by the American Academy of Pain Management and is certified by the American Society of Neurorehabilitation. He is a Senior Disability Analyst and Diplomate of the American Board of Disability Analysts and a board-certified forensic examiner. He is also a Diplomate of the American Board of Forensic Medicine.

Dr. Jay founded and was the first president of the Southern California Pain Society. He has served on the Board of Directors of the American Association for the Study of Headache (AASH). He was the Chairperson of the Professional Education group of the Brain Injury Interdisciplinary Special Interest Group, a part of the American Congress of Rehabilitation Medicine. There, he helped develop the core curriculum to be used to teach professionals about traumatic brain injury. He has been one of the presenters for the National Pain Medicine Board Review Course for 3 years and has lectured nationally for 18 years. He is Chairman of the Colorado State Department of Labor RSD/CRPS Task Force, and Co-Chair of the Chronic Pain Task Force. He has been the Medical Director of Pain and Traumatic Brain Injury Services in several hospitals over the last decade.

Dr. Jay has published over 30 medical textbook chapters and medical articles in peer-reviewed journals, all dealing with various aspects of headache, pain, and mild traumatic brain injury. He is also the author of a book dealing with headache for the lay public.

Currently, Dr. Jay is the Executive Medical Director of the Headache and Neurological Rehabilitation Institute of Colorado, P.C., in Northglenn (www.hnric.com).

Contents

Dedication

This book is dedicated to all the patients I have seen and treated for headache over the last 18 years. My warmest thanks — you have taught me more than any books could have! Even more important, it is dedicated to my incredibly smart and understanding wife, Suzanne, and my equally incredible daughter, Samantha, who will probably know all this and more by the time she is ten.

chapter one

Anatomy and physiology of headache

The diagnosis and treatment of headache should be considered a subspecialty. Why do I say this? It takes a great deal of specialized information, as well as a lot of general information, to do it right. The purpose of this book is to give to you, the interested clinician, the specialized information you may not have had a chance to collect. The information will help you diagnostically, as well as with treatment, which will be discussed in some depth. You will learn some "tricks" of the trade, as well as some common sense things which, believe me, usually are not commonly thought of in clinical practice. We will discuss patient cases and go through the thought processes used to arrive at the correct diagnosis. We will also explore treatment, both specifically and generally, as well as the neuropharmacology of the drug treatment of headache.

Occasionally we will come to an **AH HA!**. This is a point of particular importance or relevance to which you may want to pay special attention. For example:

> **AH HA!** *Just because a new patient says they have migraine headache, DO NOT take that diagnosis at face value!*

Why not take what the patient says at face value? Many patients think of all headaches as being the same thing — a pain in the head. The term "migraine" means the same thing as "headache" to most of them. Diagnostic differentiation is not their responsibility; it is yours, as a clinician. Ask the patient if the diagnosis of migraine was given by a clinician. If not, start your history again. Even if the diagnosis *was* made by a physician, start your history again anyway. Physicians and chiropractors who do not specialize in headache can be wrong. This typically leads to unsuccessful treatment of the patient for migraine, and both patient and doctor become frustrated — the patient, because his headaches are not better, and the clinician, because he knows that the treatment he administered for migraine was correct. The patient did not get better, so there must be something "wrong" with the patient. It must be the patient's fault! (But then, treating the incorrect diagnosis correctly does not help very much!) And so it goes.

When such patients finally reach someone who specializes in headache, they are angry, depressed, dismissive, and, in effect, are daring you to help them! Remember, though, an incorrect diagnosis is not the patient's fault. The patient's experience, however, will make treatment more of a challenge for you now. It is intent of this book to teach you how not to make such sophomoric mistakes and how to intervene appropriately and correctly when you are called upon to do so.

First, lets get some "words" down.

> **AH HA!** *For the remainder of this book, the terms "clinician" and "physician" are interchangeable and include both doctors of medicine and chiropractic.*

We are not here to split hairs, nor fight stupid battles. Members of both professions are equally able to utilize this information. Also, to save trees, the titles of clinicians, chiropractors, and physicians are meant to mean both male and female members of the professions. No sexism allowed. Please note, too, that all non-generic medication names are trademarked.

Now that we have that all straightened out, let's get started! This chapter will deal with the anatomy and physiology of headache. It will get pretty complex, for which we are not sorry, since that is the way the central nervous system (CNS) is built. You should be familiar with this information, as it will help you to understand (anatomically, physiologically, and, later, neuropharmacologically) some of the diagnostic and treatment aspects we will be talking about. There will be more anatomy and physiology later, too.

If you want to skip ahead to the chapters dealing with specific clinical entities, go ahead, but come back here later on and absorb what you can.

Because there has to be a place to start, we will begin with the cranial nerves — specifically, the functional components of the cranial nerves. I mean, we have to start somewhere! There are two types of general afferent fibers. Remember, afferent fibers carry information *to* the central nervous system. *General somatic afferents* (GSA) carry pain, temperature, touch, and proprioceptive information from sensory endings in the body wall, tendons, and joints. The *general visceral afferents* (GVA) carry impulses from the visceral organs within the thoracic, abdominal, and pelvic cavities. There are also special afferent fibers, including *special somatic afferents* (SSA) which carry sensory information from organs in the eye and ear for vision, hearing, and equilibrium. The *special visceral afferents* (SVA) carry olfactory and gustatory impulses.

The general efferent fibers come *from* motor neurons in the spinal cord, brainstem, and autonomic ganglia and innervate all musculature of the body, except the branchiomeric muscles. There are three types. *The general somatic efferents* (GSE) convey motor impulses to somatic skeletal muscles via fibers in the ventral roots of spinal nerves. The *general visceral efferents* (GVE) are autonomic axons which control smooth and cardiac muscle and regulate glandular secretion. The *special visceral efferent* (SVE) fibers innervate striated skeletal muscles in the jaw, the muscles of facial expression, and the muscles of the pharynx and larynx.

That being said, let's look at various aspects of the cranial nerves. The *olfactory nerve* (I) consists of SVA fibers which terminate in the olfactory bulb. The *optic nerve* (II) consists of SSA fibers which go to the evaginated fiber tract of the diencephalon, from which they continue on through relays in the thalamus (via the lateral geniculate body) to the occipital lobes.

The *oculomotor nerve* (III) contains GSA, which comes from extrinsic ocular muscles. Central processes may terminate in the trigeminal nucleus. The third cranial nerve also has general somatic efferents, fibers from the oculomotor nucleus which innervate the extrinsic muscles of the eye, except for the superior oblique and lateral rectus muscles. This cranial nerve also has preganglionic parasympathetic fibers from the accessory oculomotor nucleus (of Edinger-Westphal) and ends in the ciliary ganglion, which controls pupillary constriction and light and accommodation reflexes.

The *trochlear nerve* (IV) includes GSA, or proprioceptive fibers from the superior oblique muscles. It also carries fibers from the trochlear nucleus which innervate the superior oblique muscle of the contralateral eye. The *trigeminal nerve* (V) is as complex as it is important. It has both exteroceptive and proprioceptive afferent fibers. The former come from the skin of the face and the anterior portion of the scalp, the mucus membranes of the mouth and nasal chamber, and the dura mater of most of the cranial cavity. The proprioceptive fibers come from the muscles of mastication and other muscles innervated by the mandibular division of the Vth nerve. Fibers from both these afferent pathways end in the trigeminal nucleus. There are also efferent fibers from the motor nucleus of the Vth cranial nerve which contribute to the mandibular nerve and innervate the muscles of mastication. Pain, or nociceptive, fibers come from the face, corneas, sinuses, and mucosa of the lips, cheeks, and tongue and are carried via the Vth nerve to its sensory ganglion, known as the gasserian ganglion (also the semilunar or the trigeminal ganglion).

The *abducen* (or VIth cranial nerve) also has both afferent and efferent aspects. There are proprioceptive (afferent) fibers from the lateral rectus muscle and efferent fibers from the abducens nucleus which innervate the lateral rectus muscle. The *facial nerve* (VII) has general somatic afferent fibers from the geniculate ganglion which convey exteroceptive sensations such as pain and temperature from the external auditory meatus and the skin of the ear. It has peripheral (SVA) fibers which terminate in the anterior two thirds of the tongue. The preganglionic parasympathetic fibers (GVE) lead from the nervus intermedius. The postganglionic fibers terminate in the lacrimal glands and submandibular and sublingual salivary glands. Special efferent fibers come from the motor nucleus of the facial nerve and innervate the superficial muscles of the face and scalp, platysma, stapedius, stylohyoid, and the posterior belly of the digastric muscle.

The *vestibulocochlear nerve* (VIII, formerly the acoustic nerve) has SSA fibers, which are peripheral processes of the cochlear part of VIII that receive stimuli from hair cells in the cochlear duct and terminate in the dorsal and ventral cochlear nuclei. The vestibular part of VIII, with fibers from the vestibular ganglion, has peripheral processes which receive stimuli from hair cells of the maculae and cristae, with the central processes ending in the four vestibular nuclei in the pons and medulla.

The *glossopharyngeal nerve* (IX) has GSA peripheral fibers which convey pain and temperature from the external auditory meatus and the skin of the ear, with central processes ending in the spinal tract of the Vth cranial nerve. There are GVA fibers from the petrosal ganglion which carry general sensory input from the posterior third of the tongue and pharynx. A branch innervates the carotid sinus and carotid body. SVA fibers carry gustatory sensations from the posterior third of the tongue. GVE postganglionic fibers innervate the parotid gland. SVE fibers from the nucleus ambiguus pass through IX to innervate the stylopharyngeus muscle.

The *vagus nerve* (X) also has five different types of functional fiber types. The GSA fibers arriving at the superior ganglion convey touch, pain, and temperature from the skin of the auricle. The central processes of these cells end in the spinal nucleus of V. The GVA fibers from the inferior ganglion carry general sensations from the pharynx and larynx and from the thoracic and abdominal viscera. Central processes end in the nucleus solitarius. The SVE include fibers from the inferior ganglion which receive gustatory stimuli from the epiglottal taste buds via the internal laryngeal nerve. The GVE preganglionic parasympathetic fibers from the dorsal motor nucleus of cranial nerve X end on postganglionic neurons in the walls of the thoracic and abdominal viscera. The nucleus ambiguus sends fibers which innervate the heart. Postganglionic fibers innervate smooth muscle and cardiac muscle. SVE fibers from the nucleus ambiguus innervate the skeletal muscle in the soft palate and pharynx.

The *accessory nerve* (XI) has two divisions. The bulbar (cranial) portion has SVE fibers which supply the muscles of the sixth branchial arch of the larynx. The spinal portion has SVE fibers from the spinal accessory nucleus in the dorsal part of the anterior horn of C_2 to C_5 in the cervical cord, which exits the spinal cord through the lateral funiculus, exits the skull in association with cranial nerves IX and X, and innervates the sternocleidomastoid and trapezius muscles. The *hypoglossal nerve* (XII) has GSA proprioceptive fibers from the lingual musculature. It also contains GSE fibers from the hypoglossal nucleus which innervate the musculature of the tongue.

You made it through the really, really hard stuff! Congratulations! Now, take a deep breath, and let's move on to the special senses, all four of them.

This stuff will come into play later on when we deal with migraine auras and similar things.

The first special sense is the *acoustic system*. Acoustical stimuli pass through the middle ear, scala vestibuli, and scala tympani to Corti's organ, where hair cells are rubbed against the tectorial membrane. Excitation of the hair cells is picked up by the cochlear nerve (VIII). Fibers enter the brainstem at the lateral pons, split, and enter the dorsal and ventral cochlear nuclei. From there, fibers proceed rostrally via the nucleus of the lateral lemniscus, the inferior colliculus on the roof of the midbrain, and the medial geniculate body. The acoustic radiation goes to Heschl's gyrus on the cortex. Then, the dulcet sounds of Dr. Dre, Hootie and the boys, and even Wagner can be recognized.

The *olfactory system* comes complete with olfactory cells, which make up the olfactory filaments, which go through the cribiform plate and enter the olfactory bulb, the projections of which are the olfactory tract, which travels through the lateral olfactory striae to the uncus. The medial olfactory striae goes through the olfactory portion of the anterior commissure to the opposite olfactory bulb.

In the *optic system*, the human retina, with rods and cones, transmits impulses to the ganglion cells, whose axons form the optic nerve. From there, axons go to the optic chiasm. From the optic chiasm, optic tracts go to the lateral geniculate body, then to the posterior calcarine fissure and adjacent areas of the occipital pole. At the optic chiasm, there is a semidecussation of the optic nerves. The tracts arising on each side of the optic chiasm contain fibers from both eyes, as well as fibers from corresponding halves of each retina (right or left) to each geniculate body.

Our sense of *taste* begins with sensory cells from the taste buds on the tongue. These cells transmit one of four distinguished qualities: sweet, sour, salty, and bitter. Most taste buds are innervated by cranial nerve IX, the glossopharyngeal nerve. The facial nerve (VII) innervates the tip of the tongue, and the vagus nerve (X) sends branches to the epiglottis and larynx. From the taste fibers through the facial nerve, the geniculate ganglion sends peripheral fibers via the chorda tympani through the pterotympanic fissure to the lingual nerve of the mandibular branch of V or via the greater superficial petrossal nerve past the otic ganglion to the lingual nerve to the tip of the tongue. Taste fibers in the brainstem — from cranial nerves VII, IX, and X — go to the solitary nucleus, where the fibers appear to cross and ascend in connection with the trigeminal lemniscal fibers. The fibers then go to the arcuate nucleus of the thalamus and from there to the parietal cortex. And that's how we recognize the taste of a good steak!

So much for the general, introductory, read-it-anywhere, basic information. Now we can become a little more specific (at least in terms of headache) as we describe the pain-sensitive structures of the head. One of the most fascinating aspects of the pain-sensitive structures of the head is that the brain is not one of them, in spite of being the "receiver" of nociceptive information from the entire body. Even so, a great number of pain-sensitive structures are important in our discussions. Most of them you have already read about in the cranial nerve discussion.

In no particular order, the pain-sensitive structures of the head include the skin; fascia; muscles, periostium of the skull, and upper cervical vertebrae; scalp vessels; orbital structures and the eyeball; salivary glands; teeth and gums; ears, including the external auditory canal and the tympanic membrane; mucus membranes of the paranasal sinuses; temporomandibular joints; dura mater within the skull; and the dural blood vessels — including those of the falx cerebri and the dural venous sinuses. Now, the how, why, and where.

Sympathetic (efferent) nerves carried on the wall of the internal carotid artery, from the cervical plexus, supply the intracranial arteries and their branches at the base of the brain. Nociceptive (afferent) fibers from the intracranial cavity above the tentorium are carried by branches of the trigeminal nerve.

Pain is usually felt in the frontal, parietal, and occipital regions. Pain from below the tentorium is carried by branches of the glossopharyngeal and vagus nerves. It is perceived in the occipital region. Pain from sympathetic nerves supplying the internal carotid artery and its major branches in the brain is felt in or behind the eyes. (Attention, cluster headache fans!) Pain from the cerebral vasculature is carried by various structures. These include:

- The sympathetic nervous system (C_8, T_{1-3} via the superior cervical ganglion) and parasympathetic fibers supply the internal and external carotid arterial systems; the greater superficial petrosal branch of the facial nerve accounts for some parasympathetic contribution.
- Branches of cranial nerves III, IV, and VI supply the carotid artery to the carotid plexus.
- The vertebral artery system receives branches from cranial nerves III, V, VII, IX, XI, and XII; this innervation is unilateral in most patients.
- The scalp is supplied by branches of the external carotid arterial system.
- The trigeminal nerve innervates the superficial temporal artery and its branches; pain from the occipital artery is accessed by the branches of the upper cervical nerve roots.
- Pain from the mucus membranes of the paranasal sinuses and the periostium of the skull, as well as the teeth and gums, is mediated by the corresponding divisions of the trigeminal nerve.

The trigeminal sensory system is extremely important in the pathogenesis of headache (particularly migraine, it seems) and pain. There are three major branches and corresponding exits from the skull: the ophthalmic, which originates from the superior orbital fissure; the maxillary, from the foramen rotundum; and the mandibular, from the foramen ovale.

The afferent fibers from the three main branches converge toward the trigeminal ganglion in Meckel's cave. Afferent neurons from the trigeminal ganglion enter the pons and bifurcate into ascending branches, which end in the main sensory nucleus in the pons. The descending branches, which run in the spinal tract of the trigeminal system, end in the descending or spinal nucleus of the trigeminal system.

Different modalities of sensation are carried by a single nerve but are relayed to different sites in the brain for processing. Proprioception from the jaw muscles goes to the midbrain nucleus of cranial nerve V. Facial sensation (touch) goes to the main sensory nucleus in the pons. Pain and temperature are perceived via the descending spinal tract and nucleus of the trigeminal nerve which become continuous with the spinal aspects in the upper cervical cord.

The descending trigeminal fibers in the spinal tract are organized somatotopically, in an inverted representation of the face. This descending tract receives fibers from cranial nerves VII, IX, and X. The spinal nucleus is divided into the oral nucleus, for perceiving touch from mucus membrane in the oral cavity; the interpolar nucleus, which perceives dental pain; and the caudal nucleus, for pain and temperature sensation from the skin of the face. The spinal nucleus, rostrally, is continuous with the main sensory nucleus and caudally extends down to the C_2 level of the spinal cord.

Fibers from the main sensory nucleus are projected into the ipsilateral thalamus via the dorsal trigeminal tract to the ventral posterior medial nucleus of the thalamus, with a somatotopic representation of the face. From there, fibers go to the primary somatosensory cortex.

Ascending afferents from the caudal nucleus have branches to the brainstem reticular formation. Afferent fibers to the vagus nerve carry pain from the posterior cranial fossa, which projects into the descending tract of the trigeminal nerve and then to the contralateral thalamus and sensory cortex.

Figures 1 and 2 demonstrate the innervation of the head and neck, as well as the central connections of the trigeminal nerve. Figure 1 is for those of you who like wiring diagrams. It helps to demonstrate the complexity of what we have been talking about. Figure 2 shows important information, particularly when a physical or neurological examination is performed.

That's it — the basic science you need to understand the anatomy and physiology of the brain. Unfortunately, we have not as yet even ventured into the very important realm of neuropharmacology, which we shall be doing with some alacrity in chapters that follow. The importance of the information given here should not be ignored. It will help you answer questions extremely important to patient diagnosis — for instance, "Where is the lesion?" or "What part of the nervous system is causing the pain?" and that old favorite, "If we were to get a block (or radiofrequency coagulation or cryo [freezing] procedure), where and what should we aim for?" Well, there have been entire textbooks written about what we have covered so far.

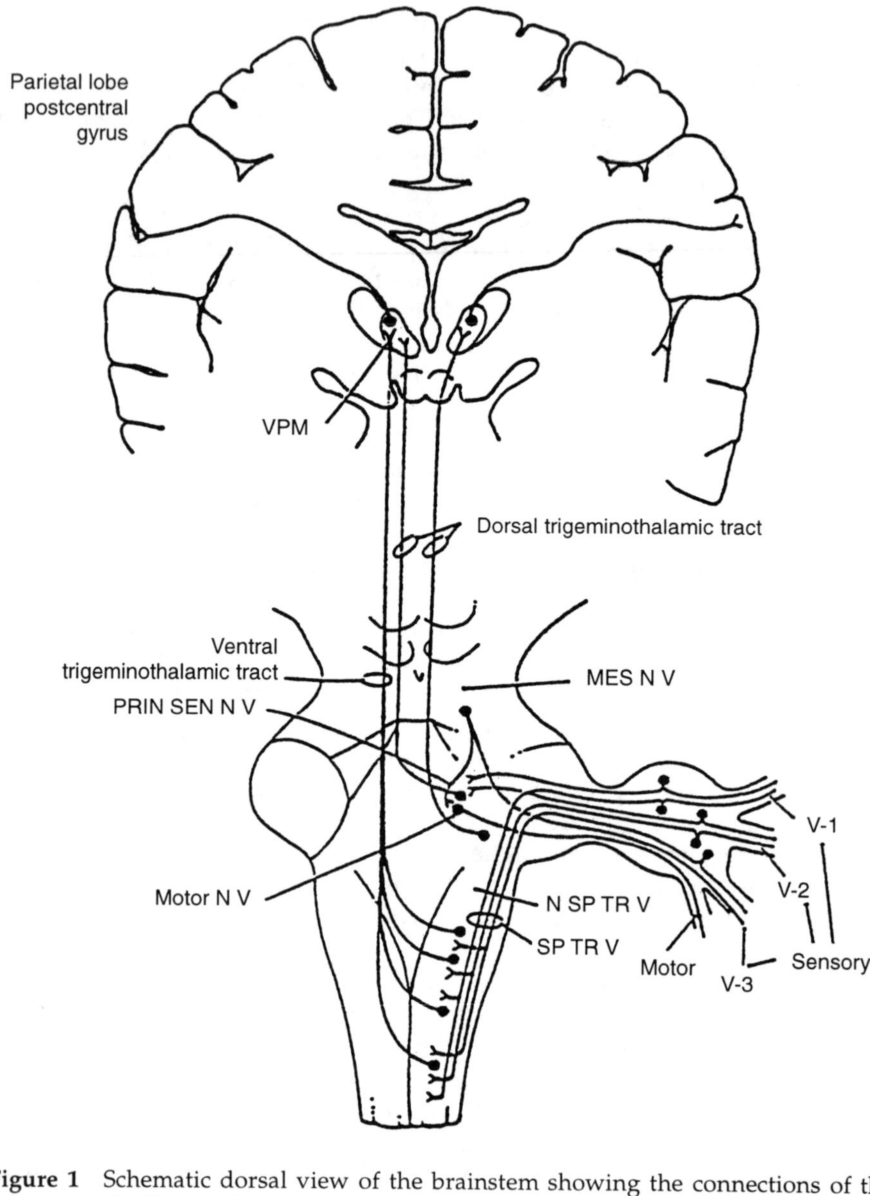

Figure 1 Schematic dorsal view of the brainstem showing the connections of the afferent and efferent fibers of the trigeminal nerve. V-1 = ophthalmic nerve; V-2 = maxillary nerve; V-3 = mandibular nerve; MES N V = mesencephalic nucleus of V; PRIN SEN V = principal sensory nucleus of V; N SP TR V = nucleus of the spinal tract of V; SP TR V = spinal tract of V; VPM = ventral posteromedial nucleus of the thalamus. (From Gilman, S. and Newman, S.W., *Manter and Gatz's Clinical Neuroanatomy and Neurophysiology*, 8th ed., F.A. Davis, Philadelphia, 1992, p. 140. With permission.)

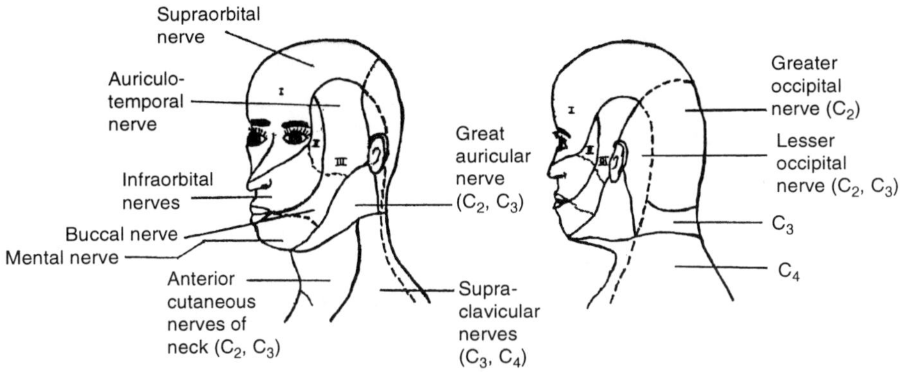

Figure 2 Innervation of the head and neck. (Adapted from Kandel, E.R. and Schwartz, J.H., *Principles of Neural Science,* Elsevier, New York, 1985, p. 563.)

Then again, we are going to go into (much) more territory where the same is also true. But, we are here for the clinical facts and procedures, not for the esoterica. Some of the information may seem esoteric, but trust me, it is not. It *will* help you!

chapter two

General thoughts on the mechanisms of headache

A bit of a breather here after last chapter's Byzantine neuroanatomy and neurophysiology. Let's extrapolate (sort of in a stream-of-consciousness way) on the problem of headache. What is the problem of headache, exactly? Your head hurts, you take some medicine, and you feel better, right? Sorry, if only it was that simple! A book like this one would not be necessary, would it?

Headache is pretty ubiquitous. Depending on whose research you read, chronic headache affects between 45 and 55 million Americans, or about 20% of the population of the United States. A further breakdown reveals that migraine affects about 18 to 20 million people; tension-type headache, almost 25 million; combination headache, at least 35 million people; cluster headache, maybe a tenth of those affected with migraine. Patients with headache secondary to brain tumors, endocrinopathies, and other medical problems are only one half of one percent of headache sufferers. That is a lot of pain, not to mention suffering!

What's the cost of headache? Well, over-the-counter drugs alone average about $4,000,000,000 a year. Prescription drugs, conservatively, probably at least double that figure. Then there is the slight problem of loss of work. How many days a year do migraine sufferers miss work because of severe headache? The days number in the millions. Multiply that by the income lost and multiply that by the costs of emergency room or physician visits (let's not count medication twice), and the costs begin to approach "billions and billions…". That is a lot of money — big time!

Now, we have not even mentioned yet the problem of suffering. And its effect on the headache sufferer's family. And friends. And co-workers. And job loss resulting from "too much time missed". And let us not forget the out-of-pocket expenses not covered by the sufferer's insurance coverage for medications, visits to clinicians, treatment, etc., *ad nauseum*.

Oh, yeah, and what about switching insurance policies and having a "pre-existing condition" that will not be covered for 6 to 12 months? And, let's not forget the exclusions on insurance policies. Some have total rehabilitation exclusions; others have *very* minimal coverage for chronic headache or pain problems, on a "life-time" basis. Would you believe one insurance company has a $2000 life-time limit for chronic headache or pain? Well, believe it. It's real. It exists.

Since we can't fight such policies, at least not now, we have to learn better care of our patients with headache. We have to find ways to make diagnoses more quickly and accurately. Treatment must be to the point and should not add to the patients' problems. How does that happen? I mean, what kind of physician would knowingly add to a patient's problems? The answer is that many good physicians do what they must in order to survive in the current state of medical "reality".

Face it. Initially, it is much easier, not to mention *cheaper*, to give pain medications to patients with pain. So, what's new? Headache specialists and other interested clinicians know that if analgesic medications are given for longer than a week or so, analgesic rebound headache can and will occur. We will go into this in much greater detail later on. But, even being aware of the drawbacks, if you work for an HMO or PPO you may be told that pain medication is the way to treat headache. Such medication, though, simply ameliorates the problem; it is palliative, not curative. But, it *is* cheap!

Now, with the continuing advent of more HMO and PPO formularies, you may not even be able to prescribe the medications you want, at least without a lot of paper shuffling to get "permission". It's true! Some formularies even deny the use of sumatriptan.

Case study

Five years ago an HMO physician sent me a patient who had a 35-year history of chronic headache. The patient was a 61-year-old gentleman who had been treated for over 30 years with analgesics. For the 10 or so years before I met the patient, he had been prescribed Fiorinal, which, as you all know, contains butalbatal, a fast-acting barbiturate, along with aspirin. This gentleman had been taking an average of 30 pills a day! Really! And it was questioned as to why should this man continue to have headache. I mean, let's get real here.

The bottom line? I physiologically weaned him off of the pain medication (slowly!) and treated him with an interdisciplinary headache rehabilitation program. Within 6 weeks, he was headache free, for the first time in over 30 years. The kicker? His HMO, which had been feeding him the barbiturates for all those years

> and a representative of which had sent the patient to see me, refused to pay for his treatment because (1) the patient was a drug addict(!) and drug "detoxification" was not covered by his policy, and (2) the rehabilitation we had completed was not covered either!
>
> It was within their medical policies to addict the man to barbiturates to treat his headaches. They essentially made him a "drug addict", but they did not want to pay for the correct treatment of his headaches, which basically involved *fixing their mistakes*!

A *Catch 22*? Yes, except the recipient of the foul ball was the patient. It took over 3 years and a great deal of time going back and forth before the HMO would pay something on the bill. Sadder still, the physician who recognized and refused to continue to be a part of the problem was reprimanded. Ya have to love it! The bean-counters strike again!

What makes this story even sadder in the re-telling is that the medical facts were there but were ignored by the HMO (which did have a "medical director"). Real and hypothetical mechanisms for headache were known 5 years ago, and many of the then hypothetical mechanisms are proving to be medically accurate and real. Let's look at these hypotheses.

Neurological

Let us assume for a moment that the problem is somewhere in the brain. Gee, I guess all the facts of the issue (or at least a lot of them) were cited in Chapter 1, but, what the hey, let's move forward and look at migraine headache, as an example. Dr. Jim Lance, from Australia, has shown that stimulation of the brainstem locus coeruleus will induce the biochemical, vascular, and physiological changes seen in "migraine". He used monkeys for his research, which deservedly won medical awards. Can't get more neurological than that, I guess.

Then there is the theory of the spreading depression of Leaõ, which for years (decades even) has been the theory of the migrainous aura. According to this theory, used to explain the visual aura of "migraine with aura" (which used to be called classical migraine), it was felt that a depression of neuronal activity began in one place and spread forward in a slow (3 to 4 mm/second) wave, or spreading depression. It would explain the facts. It has not been as well documented as Lance's work, at least not in human beings, but certainly, medically and research-wise, it appears to be real. Yes, there are other neurological examples, but let's move on for now to the next mechanism.

Serotonergic abnormalities

Serotonin, or 5-HT (5-hydroxy-tryptamine) has been determined to be a major player in the neurochemical etiology of headache. Not just for one type of headache, but for many. Changes in the serotonergic system may be seen in both acute and chronic headache and other (somatic) pain problems. Such changes do vary in ways which depend on the type of headache, as we shall see.

Decreases in serotonin are associated with a decreased pain threshold, depression, sleep abnormalities, and abnormalities of hypothalamic hormonal release. Along with the endogenous opiates, serotonin is affected by the "empty neuron syndrome" (see the chapter on tension-type headache).

The importance of serotonin in nociception can be seen in a simple experiment. Reserpine, used in the past for hypertension, eliminates the biogenic amines, of which serotonin is one. Immediately after reserpine is effective, a bolus of narcotic will not be particularly useful in ameliorating pain. Without serotonin, the endogenous opiate system is standing on one, not two, legs.

Neil Raskin, M.D., in his textbook, *Headache*, stated that headache may be the "noise" generated by changes in serotonergic tone in the central nervous system. Me, I think he is right. There are other neuropharmacological abnormalities, though.

Neuropharmacological abnormalities

Aside from serotonin, as we shall see in (perhaps nauseating) detail, the endogenous opiates, as well as norepinephrine, are affected, particularly in tension-type headache. Neuropeptide Y, acetylcholine, vasoactive intestinal peptide (VIP), calcitonin gene-related peptide (CGRP), and substance P are also involved, among others, particularly in migraine.

A host of other neuropharmacological changes are involved in headache of various types. We will learn more about these, as well as how knowing about these changes gives us a hand up in the pharmacological treatment of headache. But, before then, there is the question of blood flow abnormalities.

Blood flow abnormalities

As Wolff realized decades ago, when he began working with the ergots, migraine has been associated with vascular changes. For decades before that, if not centuries, going back to the ancient Greeks, it was a question of whether or not the vascular changes were primary or secondary. The answer is, as Lance and others have shown, that the vascular changes (such as vasodilatation and vasoconstriction) are secondary to neurological events. These vascular changes are most specifically seen in the primary vascular headaches: migraine and cluster headache.

Other questions still remain, including the existence and possible importance of cephalic arteriovenous shunts in the etiology or pathophysiology of migraine, which brings us to the burning question of myofascial mechanisms.

Myofascial mechanisms

I have lectured about the pathophysiology of myofascial mechanisms of headache on the same podium with other headache specialists who stated that, categorically, there were no such things. One of these nay-saying specialists had previously written a book on headache and included a chapter on "muscle contraction headache". So, the question is not one of reality, but of which side of the bed you get up on. Or something like that.

Myofascial (muscular) mechanisms appear to be secondary epiphenomena in migraine. In tension-type headache, these mechanisms are initially primary, then become secondary. Tension-type headache may be associated with a myofascial pain syndrome as well as fibromyalgia. These myofascial mechanisms may be insidious in origin or post-traumatic in etiology. The treatment, as well as the consequences of poor or inappropriate treatment, is the same.

So, we have now briefly visited with the basic hypothetical mechanisms of headache. We will be dealing with each primary headache type on an individual basis and will go into the up-to-date pathophysiology, as well as treatment. Again, I remind you that all of this high-falutin' stuff is great for cocktail party discussion and for playing *Jeopardy*, but the major purpose — the only reason to learn this information — is to help your patients. Now that we have had a little break, let's talk about migraine headache.

chapter three

Migraine headache

Migraine headache is an old, old problem, with mention of them going back about 5000 years. Descriptions of migraine go back to Sumeria, around 3000 BC, as well as to Mesopotamia.[3,4] Hippocrates, in 400 BC, described the visual aura.[5] Celsus, somewhere around 215 to 300 AD described triggers to migraine, including wine.[5]

Galen, in approximately 200 AD, introduced the Greek word *hemicrania* ("half head"), from which the word migraine was finally derived.[6] Tissot (1783) believed that migraine was different from a "typical" headache in that it was supraorbital neuralgia "provoked by reflexes from the stomach, gallbladder, or uterus."[6] Liveing (1873) wrote the first medical monograph on migraine — "On Megrim, Sick-Headache, and some Allied Disorders: A Contribution to the Pathology of Nerve Storms" — in which he originated the neurological theory of migraine. He felt that migraine was secondary to "nerve storms" which were "disturbances of the autonomic nervous system."[7]

For decades, the debate over the pathogenesis of migraine being neurological or vascular raged. Wolff[8] elaborated upon the vascular theory of migraine in the 1940s and 1950s. Since then, a number of physicians have continued the debate. In the 1980s, migraine settled back into a neurological theory and has remained there. Okay, so I threw in some esoterica. Enjoy it.

Some more statistics: For the period from 1977 to 1978, a medical care survey found that approximately 4% of all medical visits were for severe headache, leading to over 10 million outpatient physician visits per year. An American survey, which included 112,000 people in 40,000 households, found that 5.5 days of restricted work and activity were due to headache per 100 people per year, or a total 11,572 days.[9]

In Washington, D.C., from 1986 to 1987, 8% of men and 14% of women missed part or more of a day of work or school because of headache in the 4 weeks prior to the study interview.[10] Another study noted that headache, migraine or otherwise, may not be the only cause of such disability. It may also be caused by the drugs used to treat the headaches.[11]

Types of migraine

So, what is a migraine? In my training, I had an attending neurologist who taught that a migraine was only a migraine if the pain was unilateral; therefore, a bilateral throbbing headache could not be a migraine. Only a unilateral throbbing headache was a migraine. Unfortunately, neither statement is true. At all.

In 1988, the Headache Classification Committee of the International Headache Society (IHS) published their new classification and diagnostic criteria for headache disorders, cranial neuralgia, and facial pain in the journal *Cephalalgia*.[12] Note that the names have been changed. Common migraine is now called "migraine without aura". Classical migraine is called "migraine with aura". The aura is considered to be the neurological symptom that occurs before or at the beginning of the pain of the attack. Auras may be visual or not. (It may be difficult to identify a migraine as opposed to a tension-type headache; this will be dealt with later on, in another chapter.)

It has been noted that, at most, 30% of migraine headaches are associated with an aura.[13] A patient may have a headache without aura or an aura without headache.[14] One study showed that in a cohort of 71 migraine patients, 22.5% always had an aura, 14.1% usually had an aura, 45.1% commonly had an aura, 12.7% occasionally had an aura, and 5.6% never had an aura, over a 3-month period.[15] There is a female predominance to migraine, about 8 to 10:1. For over 80% of patients, there is a familial history of migraine.

Migraine without aura (common migraine, in the past), according to the IHS description noted above,[12] is diagnosed after at least five attacks. The duration of the headache is 4 to 72 hours in the adult, 2 to 48 hours in children. The quality of the headache must include at least two of the following: unilateral location, pulsating pain, moderate to severe intensity, and aggravation from walking stairs or simple routine physical activity. Patients must have at least one of the following: nausea and/or vomiting or photophobia and phono- or sonophobia (which is also sometimes incorrectly called hyperacusis). Neurological examination must have ruled out an organic cause of the headaches.

Diagnostically, patients who suffer from migraine with aura[12] (previously called classical migraine) must have at least two attacks which have three of four characteristics: (1) one or more reversible aura symptoms indicative of focal cerebral cortical and/or brainstem dysfunction; (2) at least one aura symptom which gradually develops over more than 4 minutes or two or more symptoms which occur in succession; (3) no aura symptom lasting more than 60 minutes (if more than one aura symptom is present, accepted duration is proportionally increased); and (4) headache following the aura with a free interval of less than 60 minutes, but which may also begin before or simultaneously with the aura. Again, there is no neurological evidence of organic disease, even after testing.

The subclassification of migraine with typical aura[12] includes all the diagnostic criteria for migraine with aura. The headache may include one or more auras, including: homonymous visual disturbance, unilateral paresthesias and/or numbness, unilateral weakness, and aphasia or unclassifiable speech difficulty. One or more of these auras may occur. They develop gradually, with a duration less than 1 hour and have complete reversibility. The most common aura is visual and may be associated with fortification spectra (zigzag lines) with scintillating edges. The fortification spectra move laterally and may leave positive or negative scotomata in their wake. Sensory aberrations are the next most common aura; these are characterized by pins and needles (paresthesias) moving along one side of the face or body. These may be accompanied by numbness, or the patient may experience only numbness. Unilateral weakness and speech problems are less common. Migraine with typical aura is now the correct nosological term. It has taken over for the older terms: ophthalmic, hemiparesthetic, or hemiparetic migraine, as well as migraine accompaniment.

Migraine with prolonged aura[12] was previously known as hemiplegic, or complicated, migraine. Familial hemiplegic migraine has a specific IHS code and is associated with a first-degree relative with identical attacks. Hemiplegic migraine is described as a migraine with one or more aura symptoms which last more than 60 minutes and less than a week. Neuroimaging is normal. The diagnostic criteria are the same as those for migraine with aura, but at least one symptom lasts more than 60 minutes but less than 7 days. Positive neuroimaging for an ischemic lesion is called migrainous infarction, regardless of symptom duration, which is typically longer than 7 days. The hemiplegia usually lasts several days but completely resolves without any residual effects. This is probably indicative of cerebral edema rather than ischemic infarction. Stroke and vasculitis must be ruled out. Hemiplegic migraine may even follow minor head trauma.[16]

Basilar migraine[12] was known as Bickerstaff's migraine, as well as basilar artery migraine. It was initially felt to affect mainly adolescent girls, but it is now known that it may affect all ages and both sexes, with the typical migrainous female predominance. Descriptively, these patients have migraine with aura. With the aura, symptoms are combinations of brainstem, cerebellar, and occipital cortex involvement. Patients experience two or more aura symptoms: visual symptoms in both the temporal and nasal fields or both eyes, typically beginning with a hemianoptic field disturbance which becomes bilateral and may lead to temporary blindness; ataxia; dysarthria; vertigo; tinnitus; bilateral paresthesias; bilateral pareses; nausea or vomiting; and changes in the level of consciousness. Diplopia, decreased hearing, nystagmus, and drop attacks may occur. Vertigo or drop attacks may occur individually with or without headache.

Ophthalmoplegic migraine[12] is described as two or more attacks of headache associated with paresis of one or more of the oculomotor cranial nerves, with no demonstrable intracranial lesion, including berry aneurysm and chronic sinusitis with a mucocele; the Tolosa-Hunt syndrome is ruled out. The diagnostic criteria include headache overlapping with paresis of one or more cranial nerves, III, IV, or VI.

The Tolosa Hunt syndrome[17] is characterized by painful ophthalmoplegia with eye pain that is steady, boring, and gnawing; involvement of nerves of the cavernous sinus; symptoms lasting days or weeks; spontaneous remission, with recurrent attacks occurring after months or years; evidence of cavernous sinus involvement on magnetic resonance imaging (MRI) or computerized axial tomography (CAT) scan; and steroid responsiveness.

Retinal migraine[12] appears to be secondary to retinal ischemia from prolonged central retinal artery constriction, which is, in fact, an aura preceding a migraine headache. It is associated with monocular scotoma or blindness lasting less than 60 minutes, with headache following within 60 minutes or even preceding the visual symptoms. Retinal migraine usually occurs in a younger person, while the typical monocular symptoms due to vascular disease — such as amaurosis fugax or TIA (transient ischemic attack) — typically occur in older people. The duration of the migrainous aura is longer than the more typical TIA. A patient with unilateral visual symptoms lasting minutes, without headache, should obtain a full neurological work up.

If you *have* to have migraine, the one to have is migraine aura without headache.[12] It may, however, scare the daylights out of you if you have no history of migraine. Episodic neurological dysfunction seen in the migrainous aura may occur without the headache. This dysfunction includes scintillating scotoma, fortification spectra, and recurrent sensory, motor, and mental phenomena. As noted above, this dysfunction may occur in patients classified as having migraine with aura. If it does, it makes diagnosis easier. If the episodic neurological dysfunction occurs alone, a full medical evaluation and long-term followup should occur. Experience shows that aura without headache is more frequent in older patients.

Speaking of older patients, migrainous accompaniments in long-lived patients were described by Fisher.[18,19] He noted that they may begin with a "flurry" of attacks after age 45. His criteria include: (1) scintillating scotoma or other visual changes (being the most typical), followed by paresthesias, aphasia, dysarthria, and paralysis; (2) build-up of the scintillations, which does not occur in cerebrovascular disease; (3) a "march" of paresthesias, which also does not occur in cerebrovascular disease; (4) a progression from one accompaniment to another, often after a delay; (5) the occurrence of two or more similar episodes, which helps to exclude embolism; (6) headache in the episode; (7) episodes lasting 15 to 25 minutes; (8) a generally benign course; (9) normal angiography that excludes thrombosis; (9) exclusion of cerebral thrombosis, dissection and embolism, epilepsy, thrombocythemia, polycythemia, and thrombotic thrombocytopenia. Fisher considered the appearance of scintillating scotoma to be diagnostic of migraine, even if they occurred without associated headache. The appearance of paresthesias, aphasia, and motor and sensory symptoms requires more of a work-up. The obvious problem is that one must rule out transient ischemic attacks. The diagnosis of transient migrainous accompaniments is one of exclusion.

There are two common migraine equivalents in children, one of which is benign paroxysmal vertigo of childhood,[20] considered to be a precursor to migraine. Episodic vertigo, which occurs for years without vestibular abnormalities on testing, should indicate a migrainous association. Possibly associated with this is the fact that frequent or constant car sickness in a child may presage the onset of migraine. Abdominal migraine is another migraine equivalent occuring mostly in children but also in adults.[21] The afflicted child may have recurring, cyclic attacks of abdominal pain with nausea and vomiting lasting 1 to 6 hours which will recede after sleep. Headache is usually absent. Also, some attacks are associated with other migrainous symptoms such as photophobia, dizziness, chills, and sweats. A family history of migraine is typically present, and most adults with abdominal migraine have a history of migraine headaches. Any migraine equivalent should be appropriately and completely worked up before final diagnosis is made.

Dysphrenic migraine or associated disturbances of cognitive function may occur in migraineurs during a migraine attack. This may include confusion and decreased concentration, either during the attack or as an aura. The mental symptoms, such as visual aura, may occur without headache (migraine aura without headache). Work-up in these cases may be substantial.

Transient global amnesia (TGA) is often a manifestation of migraine which involves the posterior cerebral circulation without associated headache. It is typically not associated with seizure activity on EEG (electroencephalography), although initially bilateral temporal lobe epilepsy was considered to be its etiology. Characteristically, these patients have retrograde amnesia for events prior to the attack and also have an inability to form new memory. There are no focal neurological signs or symptoms on examination. As noted, TGA may be accompanied by migraine headache or it may occur in the absence of a headache.

Acute confusional migraine[22,23] is typically seen in adolescence. It is associated with confusion, agitation, and disorientation which may occur with or without a headache. When a headache occurs, it is usually mild and comes on after the confusion clears, although the headache may precede the confusion. The episode of confusion may last for minutes to several hours. There is usually a family history of migraine. The confusion is thought to be due to cortical or subcortical dysfunction secondary to ischemia or edema. No epileptiform discharges are seen on testing. TGA and acute confusional migraine typically occur as a single episode in patients with migraine and rarely reoccur.

Clinical aspects of migraine

While the typical patient develops migraine between the ages of 20 and 40, it may occur earlier or later, in the fifth decade and beyond. There are five phases of migraine,[24] which include the prodrome, which occurs hours to days before the headache; the aura, which precedes the headache by 30 to 60 minutes; the headache; the headache termination; and the postdrome. A migraine may be "complete" by having all five phases, or it may have only three or four of the phases.

The prodrome may consist of emotional, cognitive, neurological, or general symptoms, such as depression, euphoria, irritability, restlessness, hyperactivity, drowsiness, and hyper- or hyposexuality. These aspects may be considered by some to be part of autonomic changes. Neurological prodromata may include photo- and phonophobia, poor concentration, episodic aphasia, and enhanced sense of smell. The general prodromal symptoms may include diarrhea, constipation, fluid retention, anorexia, food cravings, and increased urination. Prodromata may continue into the aura, headache, and postdrome aspects of the migraine attack which indicates that they are a part of, not just a prelude to, the migraine attack. The various types of aura — visual, neurologic, dysphrenic — and other phenomena have been described above. Not mentioned, however, was that visual distortions and hallucinations may be types of visual auras.

The headache itself typically ranges from moderate to severe or even incapacitating in severity. It is usually unilateral but may be bilateral; it may remain on the same side or alternate at various times. The pain is described most often as throbbing and is associated with nausea, vomiting, photophobia, and phonophobia. As physical activity increases the pain, patients with migraine prefer to lie in a dark, quiet room. The headache may occur at any time. It is not brought on by stress but does occur after a stressful period. The pain usually builds gradually and then recedes. In the adult, the headache will last from 4 to 72 hours, 2 to 48 hours in children. Most patients have one to four attacks of migraine a month, with ranges from one per year to five to six per month in the extreme.

The migraine headache is also typically associated with skin pallor, mood changes, and hypertension, as well as hypotension and bradycardia — again, mostly autonomic nervous system signs and symptoms. Other associated symptoms may include cervical pain, peripheral edema (which can begin during the prodrome), and scalp muscle and masseter tenderness.

The headache winds down, without a specific point of termination. The postdrome is likened to a hangover. Patients may feel tired and irritable and may exhibit impaired concentration, muscle weakness and aching, and anorexia.

Migraine triggers

Migraine is known to be triggered by environmental, psychological, neurochemical, and neuroendocrine changes. This, it must be remembered, is in contradistinction to aspects of migraine prodrome, such as depression, anxiety, and even chocolate cravings. The most common migraine trigger is diet. The "big four" provocative substances include red wine and other alcoholic beverages; aged, sharp cheddar cheese (tyramine); phenylethylamine from chocolate (in few patients, as eating chocolate is now thought to be part of the prodrome); and estrogenic birth control pills. Nitrates, nitrites, milk/cheese/dairy products, eggs, fatty foods, and food additives are also felt to contribute to the problem.

Is the problem food allergy? Research is leaning heavily towards a big "no". That is, there is no true allergic response to any food, as identified by an increase in the body's immunological system, including IG_E production. A patient's ability or inability to metabolize certain substances, though, may start a neurochemical cascade which triggers a migraine.

Other triggers include hunger, sleeping too much or too little, jet lag, high altitude, barometric changes, post-stress or let-down situations, glaring lights, pungent odors, exercise (including sexual activity), head trauma, and hormonal factors.

The question of hormonal migraine is important. Before puberty, there is no statistical differentiation between male and female migraineurs. The female predominance begins after puberty and appears to be secondary to estrogenic changes, as the typical menstrual migraine occurs before, during, or after menstruation or at ovulation. It is during these times that there is the greatest fluctuation (downward) of estrogen levels. The headaches may then be secondary to "estrogen withdrawal" in susceptible women.

Pregnant women may experience an increase in migraine during the first trimester. Though many women become headache free during the later trimesters, about 25% have no changes in their headaches. Menstrual migraine patients typically improve with increased, sustained estrogen levels. While migraine is said to diminish or stop in about two thirds of women at menopause, it can worsen or remain unchanged. In rare instances, migraine may begin after menopause.

The use of estrogenic birth control pills can induce migraine most often in patients with a family history of migraine. It may exacerbate present migraine, but in some cases patients' migraine headaches improve. A major question has been the risk of stroke in migrainous women taking birth control pills. One large study found that it was migraine itself, not the birth control pills, which increased the risk for stoke.[25]

Unfortunately, when I first began my practice I worked with a 25-year-old nurse with migraine who was taking estrogenic birth control pills. She also smoked cigarettes. She sustained a "minor stroke" which caused persistent quadrantanopsia. She never regained the sight in the areas affected.

It may be a threefold problem, then: migrainous women on estrogenic birth control pills who smoke may experience an increased incidence of stroke, compared to otherwise healthy patients. To be on the safe side, I will not treat a woman with migraine on birth control pills who insists on continuing to smoke after I have explained the possible problems. While some other headache specialists may disagree with my stand, I have seen the results, rare though they may be, and I do not want to risk a patient's health.

It should be remembered that not all migraine patients are susceptible to the same triggers; in others, no triggers can be identified.

> **AH HA!** *As an important aside, when dealing with patients who have experienced their first migraine headaches, care must be taken in diagnosis to rule out other causes. For a patient whose first headache began during exercise (thunderclap headache), you must rule out organic causes such as dissecting or blown cerebral aneurysm, "signal" subarachnoid hemorrhage or leakage, and so on. Other warning signs may include changes in cognition or consciousness, stiff neck, neurological signs of subarachnoid hemorrhage, fever, and focal neurological findings.*

Pathophysiology of migraine

Migraine appears to be a hereditary perturbation of serotonergic neurotransmission. Patients with this serotonergic dysmodulation who are subjected to excessive afferent input, possible changes in neurochemical milieu, or hormonal or otherwise related internal clock changes may develop a vascular headache.

The cortex and hypothalamus operate on the brainstem to produce changes in micro- and macrocirculation via fibers from both the serotonergic system (the serotonergic nucleus raphe magnus is directly "connected" to the hypothalamus) and the noradrenergic system (via the locus coeruleus), which are distributed through the brain and terminate diffusely in the cortex near vessels of microcirculation. As noted before, stimulation of the primate locus coeruleus induces the vascular and neurochemical changes seen in migraine.

Ischemia of the occipital cortex secondary to activity of the locus coeruleus (LC) may produce the visual aura via a relative oligemia from the spreading depression of Leaõ. This phenomenon has been well established in experimental situations but is thought to be analogous to the human aura. Subsequent release of the endogenous pain-control system facilitates headache (usually one-sided), but pain may occasionally be referred to the neck and the upper quadrant of the body and even down the leg.

Pain pathways for headache perception pass through the trigeminal ganglion and the dorsal root ganglion at C_2. Neurotransmission in this pathway is modulated from the periaquaductal gray (PAG) area and the locus coeruleus.

The trigeminovascular system appears to be the main pathway for the pain of migraine. Neurophysiological changes such as the spreading depression of Leaõ induce release of nociceptive substances from the neocortex into the interstitial spaces. Within the perivascular space, these released nociceptive substances activate and sensitize the trigeminovascular fibers surrounding pial vessels and cause impulses to be conveyed to the trigeminal nucleus caudalis and then more rostrally. It is also possible that neurochemicals which are released from the cortex may stimulate menengeal vessels, which in turn release nociceptive substances.[26]

Other important facts are known. Regional blood flow studies demonstrate a unilateral reduction in cerebral blood flow during migraine with aura, inducing a period of oligemia which is followed by a period of hyperemia, probably reflexive.[27] In migraine without aura, changes in blood flow are still undetermined. EEG studies in migraine patients reveal only nonspecific changes, which may reflect only minor dysfunction secondary to spreading oligemia.[28] Other studies have identified additional abnormalities in children with migraine.[29]

A great deal of evidence has shown the changes in serotonin associated with migraine. During the aura phase and the first part of the headache, plasma serotonin levels abruptly rise; this is followed by an excess of the serotonin metabolite 5-hydroxyindoleacetic acid in urine.[30] A significant drop in levels of platelet serotonin during migraine headache has also been noted.[31]

Symptoms reflecting increased excitability in the trigeminal system have been noted. It is common for migrainous patients to experience sudden pain on ingesting ice cream (ice cream headache),[32] as well as sudden jabs of pain in the head called "ice-pick pains".[33] Both are most commonly felt on the typical side of the headache.

One important piece of evidence of the central nervous system association was published by Raskin, Hosobuchi, and Lamb[34] and Weiller, et al.,[35] who showed that in patients without a history of migraine, the disorder may arise after deep electrode stimulation for pain, of the periaquaductal gray and the nucleus raphe magnus (NRM).

Migraine also appears to be associated with vasodilator neuropeptides which are released in response to trigeminal activation. These include calcitonin gene-related peptide (CGRP) and vasoactive intestinal peptide (VIP). Electrical stimulation of the trigeminal ganglion in humans leads to an increase in extracerebral blood flow and to the release of both CGRP and substance P. Similar stimulation in cats shows release of VIP.

As noted above, the dorsal raphe nucleus (DRN) is serotonergic and receives input from the hypothalamus. The locus coeruleus (LC) is noradrenergic. Activation of these nuclei would be expected to produce vascular responses, with the LC producing vasoconstriction and the DRN producing vasodilatation. The dorsal raphe nucleus and locus coeruleus are also closely associated with the reticular formation, which "correlates" or integrates the information from these systems, and others both rostrally and caudally.[36]

It appears that parasympathetic projections from the brainstem regions which contain acetylcholine and VIP innervate intracranial meningeal blood vessels through the ipsilateral first division (ophthalmic) of the trigeminal ganglion. Activation of these pathways may release nitric oxide (NO), which is a potent vasodilator and induces, along with neurokinin A, neurovascular extravasation, creating a vicious cycle of vasodilatation and pain.[37–40]

If there is a migraine pain "generator", it appears that it may be the trigeminal nucleus caudalis.[41] Pseudo-unipolar trigeminal neurons provide sensory innervation to extracerebral, intracranial blood vessels; they also have central projections which end behind the blood-brain barrier within the trigeminal nuclei, which extend from the caudal medulla to the upper cervical spinal cord.[42] This may provide a pathway for nociception from the meningeal vessels to the central nervous system.[43] The ascending trigeminothalamic tract, which arises from the trigeminal nuclei, transmits pain impulses to the reticular formation which then go rostrally to the thalamus and continue on to the cortex.[44] Understanding this allows a more concise explanation of migraine headache.

Many of the prodromal aspects of migraine are autonomic in nature. It may be appropriate to suggest that the hypothalamic projections to the brainstem initiate extracranial vasodilatation and intracranial vasoconstriction through the LC and the DRN. Contralateral inhibition at the LC, DRN, or spinal trigeminal nucleus would then make the vasodilatation and trigeminovascular reflex predominate unilaterally, causing one-sided headache.

It should also be remembered that the release of neuropeptides (as noted above) may augment the action of monoamine neurotransmitters, such as serotonin, and induce a sterile perivascular inflammation (a point which is no longer well accepted), as well as helping in the sensitization of intracranial blood vessels. The vessels respond to vasodilatation by increasing afferent nociceptive discharges, which would seem to increase the activity of brainstem nuclei, helping to perpetuate a vicious neurochemical and neurophysiological cycle, the migraine.

Therapy

Pharmacological treatment of migraine is of two types — abortive and prophylactic. The abortive therapies tell us the most about treatment as well as about the pathophysiology of migraine.

There are at least 14 subtypes of specific serotonergic receptors in the central nervous system, with seven subfamilies.[45] The most important for our discussion are the 5-HT $(\text{serotonin})_{1A}$ and 5-HT_{1D} receptors. Both of these receptor subtypes cause neuronal inhibition of central nervous system neurons, as well as cause contraction of some vascular smooth muscle.

The 5-HT_{1D} receptors are present in the intracranial blood vessels and are the most common receptor subtype in the human brain. The 5-HT_2 receptors induce vasoconstriction of most blood vessels and bronchospasm and contraction of the gastrointestinal smooth muscle. It therefore stands to reason that for acute treatment, we need to provide agonist activity at the 5-HT_{1A} and 5-HT_{1D} receptors, while antagonistic activity at the 5-HT_2 receptors will give us prophylactic properties.

Until now, sumatriptan has been the most potent and selective 5-HT_{1D} receptor agonist. It is five times less potent at the 5-HT_{1A} receptors and is inactive at other neurotransmitter binding sites. There are at least a half dozen or so other triptans being developed. They are mostly differentiated by their bioavailability or their serum half-lives and whether or not they can affect the central brainstem "migraine pain generator". Some studies have shown that "brain penetrant" serotonin agonists inhibit the response of the trigeminal nucleus caudalis to nociceptive stimulation.[46,47]

While all triptans will act essentially the same way — via vasoconstriction of pain-producing meningeal vessels, inhibition of peripheral trigeminal nerves, and inhibition of nociceptive activity in the brainstem trigeminal sensory nuclei — their abilities to perform central inhibition as well as their half-lives and bioavailability are important.

Dihydroergotamine (DHE-45), an ergot, is most potent at the 5-HT_{1A} receptors. It has a high affinity for $alpha_1$ and $alpha_2$ adrenergic receptors and a moderate or greater affinity for 5-HT_{1C}, 5-HT_2, and $dopamine_2$ receptors in the brain. It may be given intravenously, intramuscularly, and intranasally.

There are major differences between triptans and DHE, however. Essentially, a triptan is like a 38-caliber bullet going to one target, while the DHE is like a blast from a shotgun shell striking multiple targets. Neuropharmacologically, this would make DHE a "dirty drug" because of its widespread neurochemical affinity to multiple types of receptor sites, as opposed to a more selective neurotransmitter receptor profile.

Both drugs do work, however. There are several ways in which these two medications appear to work their anti-migraine effects. Neuronally, 5-HT_{1D} receptors appear to modulate neurotransmitter release. The efficacy of 5-HT_{1D} agonists (including DHE) may be in antagonizing endogenous transmitter release. On a vascular basis, 5-HT_{1D} receptors have been implicated in the constriction of arteriovenous anastomoses. Both triptans and DHE are probably able to block the development of neurogenic plasma extravasation of nociceptive agents, thus effectively blocking the initiators of nociceptive impulses. Both also induce vasoconstriction of meningeal vessels. Do not forget that triptans should not be given within 24 hours of any ergot, including DHE, and visa versa.

The treatment of an acute migraine may take many forms. It should be remembered that during the migraine, there is decreased absorption of oral medications secondary to decreased gastric functioning. Intravenous metaclopramide (which can induce an extrapyramidal reaction) is very useful in helping to decrease nausea and vomiting, and it promotes vascular emptying. It is typically given about 30 minutes before an oral drug, in doses of 10 to 20 mg. Other antiemetics frequently used include chlorpromazine, promethazine, hydroxyzine, and prochlorperazine. Parenteral (intravenous or intramuscular) administration or rectal suppository is best when using these agents adjunctively with narcotics.

Most patients have already tried aspirin and acetaminophen many times before coming to the physician asking for something "stronger". Narcotic analgesics may be useful in helping patients who are unable to tolerate vasoconstrictors. Combination drugs, such as butalbatal with aspirin or acetaminophen, may be useful if used sparingly. Oxycodone and hydrocodone bitartrate are stronger than codeine and meperidine when used orally.

Nonsteroidal antiinflammatory drugs (NSAIDs) may be useful in acute migraine, specifically the faster-acting agents such as IM ketorolac, 60 mg. This medication has been used frequently with DHE-45 and meperidine. Meclofenamate sodium, 200 mg at the onset of headache and 100 to 200 mg in an hour, has been shown to be useful. Naproxen, naproxen sodium, and ibuprofen are more effective than placebo. An NSAID may be used with ergotamine tartrate.

Ergotamine tartrate may be utilized orally, rectally, or sublingually. Caffeine is added to the oral or rectal forms. It is best utilized rectally, but this is most inconvenient. Ergotamine tartrate is a very potent vasoconstrictor which specifically affects the external carotid system and reportedly has no significant intracranial vasoconstrictive effects. It is contraindicated in patients with liver disease, ischemic disease, and chronic illness. It reduces neurogenic (sterile) inflammation in the dura mater and has central effects on serotonin metabolism. The most common side effects are nausea and vomiting, found in 40 to 50% of patients. Diarrhea, tingling in the extremities, and muscle cramping are also seen. Rare patients with extreme sensitivity to the drug may experience chest pain and tingling in the extremities.

The use of ergotamine tartrate is typically routine. One or two 1-mg tablets are taken at the onset of the migraine attack, and one is repeated in one-half-hour increments for two or three additional doses, if needed. The 2-mg suppository is used at the onset of the attack and once more, in one hour, if needed. One of the 2-mg sublingual tablets is taken at the onset, and one more in an hour, if needed. A bitter taste is often associated with its use, which may result in poor patient compliance.

The major problem with the use of ergotamine tartrate is over-utilization. It should be used no more than once every 7 days to prevent vascular rebound headache. This frequency is less than that indicated in the *Physicians' Desk Reference*, but clinical experience has shown this schedule to be better than more frequent usage. If a patient has a migraine more frequently than weekly, prophylactic agents should be used.

Isometheptene mucate is a mild vasoconstrictive agent with fewer side effects than ergotamine tartrate. It is therefore better tolerated. Two capsules are taken at the onset of the headache, followed by one or two more capsules in an hour, a dose which may be repeated again in one hour. It usually is combined with acetaminophen.

We have discussed DHE-45 above. It should be used intravenously, 30 minutes or so after administering 10 mg metaclopramide, also intravenously. The dosage of DHE-45 is between .5 and 1 mg, which may be repeated in about an hour. It is also effective when used intranasally. Some clinicians have patients self-inject DHE-45 two or three times a day for several weeks. This is a bad idea, as the pharmacokinetics differ so greatly in different people via an IM route. I have also seen far too many sterile abscesses. The intranasal use of DHE has been well thought out and may be useful for the patients who do not benefit from a triptan.

Sumatriptan was also discussed above. As noted, it decreases nausea and vomiting (especially when used subcutaneously). The subcutaneous injection is 6 mg and typically produces relief within less than an hour. Another injection may be given at that time if needed. Side effects may include short-lived symptoms of warmth, flushing, a pressure-like feeling in the chest, and irritation at the injection site. Not infrequently, patients who obtain relief from this medication may develop a reoccurrence of headache within 24 hours. Typically, another injection is taken. In a good number of patients, there is less possibility of the recurrent headache if the second dose is given one hour after the first, even if the patient is headache free at that time. There is also an oral form of sumatriptan; a 50-mg tablet may be taken at the onset of the headache and repeated in one hour. Relief is much slower than from the subcutaneous injection. Nausea and vomiting may last longer. An intranasal preparation is also available.

A subject of some debate is the question of sumatriptan rebound headache. I have seen it numerous times in patients using the medication more frequently than once every week to 10 days. Other headache specialists have reported seeing the same phenomenon. The new triptans are, at this time, all given orally, but they have not been on the market long enough to have as much information about them as we do for sumatriptan. As previously noted, there are at least five or six more triptans in the pipeline at this time.

Phenothiazines such as chlorpromazine and prochlorperazine used intravenously have been reported to abort acute migraine headache. The latter drug is probably safer. Care should be taken to watch for an acute extrapyramidal episode, as well as hypotension.

The use of corticosteroids for an acute attack is rare. They may be used for migraine which will not break, after one or two days. Dexamethasone, 1.5 mg twice a day for 2 or 3 days, may be helpful. Parenterally, methylprednisolone acetate, 40 to 80 mg, may be used. Parenteral corticosteroids are most useful in aborting a prolonged migraine attack. "Status migrainosus" is a migraine headache lasting longer than 72 hours. These patients are usually dehydrated from constant vomiting, and may have an electrolyte imbalance. Long-acting dexamethasone (12 to 16 mg) or methylprednisolone (40 to 80 mg) is given intramuscularly, along with sedatives and antiemetics and intravenous hydration. Repetitive intravenous DHE-45, .5 to 1 mg given every 8 hours for six to eight doses, is also helpful.

Prophylactic medication therapy should be used when patients have two or more migraine headaches a month (some believe it should be used for three or more headaches a month). The degree of disability brought on by a single headache as well as the intensity and duration are also part of the decision. If a patient has difficulties with abortive therapy, prophylactic treatment should be started.

Now go back several pages to the discussion of serotonin receptors. 5-HT_2 receptor antagonists are utilized for prophylaxis. These include the serotonergic drug methysergide. Using methysergide more than 5 months in a row may bring on serious side effects such as retroperitoneal fibrosis. The drug is started at 2 mg a day and increased to one 2-mg tablet taken two to three times a day. It is imperative to stay alert for possible side effects.

The tricyclics, doxepin and amitriptyline, are 5-HT_2 antagonists, although there is a question as to whether they work more by blockade of serotonin uptake. At one point, the use of amitriptyline was touted as a good migraine prophylactic, but at 50 to 200 mg a day its anticholinergic side effects were significant. The specific serotonin re-uptake inhibitors (SSRIs) may be helpful.

Cyproheptadine, an antihistamine with mild to moderate antiserotonin effects, is best used for children with migraine. It is well tolerated, with some side effects including increased appetite, weight gain, sedation, and dry mouth. It is given 8 to 16 mg a day in two to four divided doses.

The calcium channel blockers (CCBs) include verapamil and nifedipine, both of which have moderate affinity for the 5-HT_2 receptors. Calcium channel blockers act on vascular smooth muscle.

Verapamil, a prototypical CCB, dilates previously constricted arteries and can therefore improve cerebral blood flow. It also has blocking effects to $alpha_2$ and $beta_2$ adrenergic receptors. Alpha adrenergic effects include modulation of neurotransmitters in cerebral synapses, with increases of norepinephrine release in the hypothalamus. It inhibits binding to D_2 dopamine receptors, as does ergotamine tartrate, which may increase serum prolactin levels. Verapamil decreases serotonin release in the brain and blocks platelet serotonin uptake and release. It is typically given in doses of 240 to 360 mg a day. The time release form, at 240 mg a tablet, may be given once or twice a day. Side effects include constipation, gastrointestinal upset, limb numbness, and gynecomastia. It is contraindicated in patients with congestive heart failure and AV conduction disturbances. Nifedipine, also a CCB, is used at doses of 30 to 120 mg per day in three divided doses. Hypotension, edema, headache, and gastrointestinal upset are common side effects.

The CCB flunarizine inhibits intracellular calcium overload. It has been found to inhibit spreading depression in animals. It reduces the release of dopamine and the metenkephalins in the corpus striatum. Flunarizine may induce the extrapyramidal syndrome, as well as depression and increased prolactin levels. It is utilized in 5- or 10-mg dosages at night for prophylaxis, or 10 to 20 mg are given intravenously or sublingually for acute migraine attacks.

A particularly helpful NSAID for prophylaxis of menstrual migraine is naproxen sodium, which is given 550 mg twice a day, starting a week before the menstrual period and through the menses. The major side effect has been gastrointestinal upset. Fenoprofen and ketoprofen also have been used for prophylaxis. The former is given at 600 mg a day, the latter 130 to 300 mg in three to four divided doses. Both of these drugs have been associated with renal difficulties, including impaired renal function and renal failure.

Valproic acid, an anticonvulsant, has recently been approved by the Food and Drug Administration (FDA) for prophylactic use in migraine. Its method of action is hypothesized to involve the GABA (gamma-aminobutyric acid, an inhibitory neurotransmitter) system. It is given at 250 mg two to three times a day. Blood work evaluating the CBC as well as liver functions should be taken initially and repeated, along with valproic acid levels, monthly for 2 or 3 months, then every 6 months. Side effects include slight weight gain and drowsiness. It may induce hepatic toxicity which is reversible. Gastrointestinal upset is frequent and is helped by using the enteric coated form of the medication.

There are also non-pharmacological treatments of migraine, such as biofeedback and psychological management, both of which complement each other. Thermal biofeedback, stress reduction, and relaxation techniques are the easiest for patients to learn and implement. Cognitive strategies in the hands of an experienced psychotherapist are also useful. Likewise, a biofeedback therapist should be both experienced and have appropriate professional training.

So, that's migraine?

Yes, that is migraine — and only migraine — seen and diagnosed and treated in its "pure" form, which is rare. The majority of patients seen in a headache clinic have several types of headache, of which migraine is only one (we will have a chapter dealing with combination headache later on in this book). The differential diagnosis of migraine may seem easy, but as always there are problems. The first rule is always to do a thorough neurological examination and what ever ancillary tests you may deem necessary on the basis of your history and examination.

> **AH HA!** *The diagnosis of headache, including migraine, is made 98% of the time from history. Many facilities utilize multiple tests to come to a diagnosis that should have been obvious if their personnel truly knew headache. Some headache clinics give all patients an EEG, MMPI, doppler blood flow studies, electroencephalogram, and facial thermograms, among other tests. These tests do nothing but pad the physician's pocket, especially when they are done even before a neurological examination shows a reason for such very specific testing.*

Once you have placed a patient on medication, you should see them more frequently for the first several months to make certain there are no significant side effects. Once you and the patient are comfortable, seeing the patient every 4 to 6 months is fine, barring other problems or new complaints. If the patient complains of increasing frequency of headache, you should completely re-evaluate them.

Some literature indicates that episodic migraine will "transform" into daily headache. This typically happens due to the addition of other, iatrogenic forms of headache or through missed diagnoses. The idea of episodic migraine transforming into daily headache, or tension-type headache, does not fit into the facts as we know them, as the neurochemical substrates are different, particularly the acute and chronic serotonergic system changes.

The over-utilization of analgesic medications, even simple analgesics such as aspirin or acetaminophen, can induce analgesic rebound headache. Too frequent usage of vasoconstrictor medications can induce vascular rebound headache.

The *Physicians' Desk Reference*, as already noted, is far more liberal at dispensing vasoconstrictor medications than one should do clinically. I have had patients who have taken ergotamine preparations daily for years. One, a truck driver, took four ergot rectal suppositories a day for over 20 years. Another patient, an accountant, was taking sumatriptan daily for over a year when I first saw him. Either common sense was not used or the physicians had no idea of how the medications worked or why.

Another common problem is that unilateral acute cervical strain/sprain may induce a one-sided headache with throbbing pain along with nausea and vomiting, photophobia, and phonophobia. This has been diagnosed as a migraine (unilateral headache with throbbing pain, etc.) and treated as such. The patient received no help, but did get vascular rebound headache. A major problem is that truly thorough examinations are not being done, or the musculoskeletal aspects were missed along with the diagnosis. Anyway, there will be more about this problem in the chapter on tension-type headache.

The best thing you can do for your patients is to provide a correct diagnosis of their headache problems early and to treat them appropriately and quickly. A way to evaluate what type of headaches patients may be experiencing is to give them blank "headache calendars" and have them indicate on it the day(s) they get headaches, the duration and intensity of each attack, any association with their menstrual cycles or ovulation, and any triggers that they can recognize (lack of sleep, red wine, etc.). Most importantly, have the patients bring their calendars with them when they see you. Then, go over the calendar in detail with your patient. That's a history! And that really helps with diagnosis.

Next we will deal with the second primary vascular headache, cluster headache. You can't miss that one!

chapter four

Cluster headache

One of my female patients with migraine gleefully described cluster headache, with which her husband had just been diagnosed, as "God's revenge on men for women having migraine." Indeed, it may feel that way, in that, by all reports, cluster headache is more painful than migraine, even to the point of patients attempting suicide to stop their headache pain. Some unfortunate patients who have had the misfortune of having both problems describe cluster headache pain as being worse than the pain of renal colic.

Romberg,[48] in 1840, gave the first description of cluster headache. Ekbom,[49] in 1947, noted the periodicity of the problem, and Kunkle et al.,[50] in 1954, noted the "clustering" pattern, terminology which gave rise to the current term, cluster headache.

The two main types of cluster headache are episodic and chronic, the latter having both primary and secondary forms. Episodic cluster headache is most common, affecting at least 80% of the cluster population. It is characterized by cluster periods which last between 1 and 5 months. Each period is followed by a symptom-free remission period of 6 to 24 months, averaging one year.

Chronic cluster headache is characterized by the absence of a remission period for at least one year. Associated with this is an increased attack frequency and greater resistance to treatment. Patients who begin having cluster headaches and never experience a remission are termed primary chronic cluster headache patients. Patients who begin as episodic cluster and then develop shorter and shorter remission periods, until they have none, are termed secondary chronic cluster patients.

Clinical aspects

The incidence of cluster headache among men is felt to be between .4 and 1%. It is primarily a male disorder, with a male-to-female ratio varying between 4.5 and 6.7 to 1. The age of onset is typically between 20 and 30, although children and older adults also develop the disorder. There is no ethnic differentiation; however, an over-representation of African Americans with cluster headache has been noted.[51,52]

The cluster headache attack may be preceded by an emotional prodrome, such as hypomania or euphoria. These changes may not be noted by the patient or may not be present. The attack itself may begin with neck pressure, unilateral or bilateral. Some patients may experience a warmth over the ipsilateral temporal region for several minutes before the attack. Mild pain may occur around the eye or temple, ipsilaterally. This may be associated with nasal stuffiness. Throbbing pain of increasing intensity may "stab" the patient in the temple, teeth, or face before settling behind the eye. The ipsilateral "stuffed" nostril may now suddenly begin to exhibit clear discharge. At its worst, numerous patients have described the pain as boring and state that, "It feels like there is someone in my head, behind my eye, trying to push it out with a hot poker." The patient may develop ipsilateral lacrimation, redness of the conjunctiva, ptosis, and miosis.

Unlike migraine patients who prefer to lie in a quiet, dark room, many cluster patients may become agitated to the point of violence. They may pace the floors, strike their head into the wall, or assail the wall with their fists. The peak intensity of pain may last from 10 to 60 minutes and gradually decrease. The typical patient experiences from one to ten headaches a day, with most experiencing one to three per day. The average duration of the attack is 45 minutes, but it may be shorter or last as long as 3 hours. Longer attacks may indicate that the diagnosis should be reviewed. The attacks occur most often after working hours. The next most common time is 90 to 120 minutes after the patient has fallen asleep, during the first rapid eye movement (REM) stage of sleep.

The pain of a cluster headache is mostly seen over the oculofrontal or oculotemporal regions, unilaterally. The pain, in episodic cluster, is typically milder at the beginning and the end of the cluster cycle. Between 70 and 85% of patients exhibit ipsilateral lacrimation or nasal stuffiness, rhinorrhea, and conjunctival redness. The partial Horner's syndrome (ipsilateral ptosis and miosis) is seen in 60 to 70% of patients. It may become permanent in .5 to 6.7% of patients.[53]

Cluster headaches may be provoked, during the cluster period, by vasodilators including nitroglycerin, alcohol, and histamine. Hypoxemia may also induce a headache. Changes in diurnal cycle and during periods following extreme stress may begin the cluster cycle. One study[54] found that the frequency of cluster periods was related to seasonal photoperiod changes (length of daylight), with the cluster periods increasing during shortening or lengthening photoperiods. The peak in cluster periods began within 2 weeks following the shortest and longest days of the year (typically July and January) and decreased within 2 weeks after daylight savings and standard time changes. While rare, it is possible for an episodic cluster patient to have an isolated cluster headache attack during their remission period. There is, as yet, no compelling evidence of a genetic predisposition to cluster headache.

Because of the sometimes idiosyncratic forms of the cluster headache, as well as the greatly smaller number of women with cluster, it may be a challenge to diagnose a woman with cluster headache. One reason is the frequent incidence of migraine. Differential diagnosis, aside from migraine, includes trigeminal neuralgia, pheochromocytoma, Raeder's syndrome, and temporal arteritis. Chronic paroxysmal hemicrania (CPH), which will be discussed later in this chapter, is another disorder to be explored.

Pathophysiology of cluster headache

Neuroendocrine changes have been found in cluster patients during their active cycle, including decreased plasma testosterone and luteinizing hormone (LH), which is possibly indicative of a hypothalamic-pituitary axis change,[55,56] and a decreased thyrotropin response to thyrotropin-releasing hormone.[57] The alteration or loss of the circadian rhythmicity of neuroendocrine substances was reported.[58,59] Several authors found decreased melatonin levels during the night during cluster periods.[60,61] Also, during cluster periods, loss of normal circadian rhythm for blood pressure and temperature,[62] beta-endorphins,[63] and plasma cortisol[61] have been found.

Impairment of sympathetic activity has been found, as demonstrated by pupillometric studies indicating a diminished response to tyramine instillation into the eye, indicative of impaired sympathetic neuronal transmission on the ipsilateral side.[64] Disturbance of the sympathetic nervous system on the side of active cluster patients was also indicated by the facial thermographic studies showing ipsilateral "cold spots" on the forehead of cluster patients between attacks as well as during cluster attacks. This suggests changes in supraorbital artery hemodynamics possibly associated with impairment of autonomic regulation.

Relative hypoxia which is uncompensated may be secondary to blunted chemoreceptor response. A relationship between cluster headache and sleep apnea-induced hypoxemia was noted,[65] with indications that the gross magnitude of hypoxemia was probably not as important as the duration of relative hypoxemia. Another study indicated that, once induced, persistent hypoxemia may be secondary to an impairment of compensatory chemoreceptor autoregulation, a condition inherent to the cluster headache period.[66]

Vasomotor changes have been noted to be indicative of an impairment in autoregulatory responses,[67] with increased cerebral blood flow noted in the external carotid artery,[68] dilation of the ipsilateral ophthalmic artery,[69] and increased cerebral blood flow during attacks.[70] The internal carotid artery was found to be narrowed during a cluster attack,[71] which may also help explain the partial Horner's syndrome via compression of the oculosympathetic nerves within the bony canal through which the internal carotid artery travels.

Neurochemically, histamine was reported to be a mediator of cluster headache.[72–74] This has been both corroborated[75,76] and denied by other authors.[77,78] It has been suggested that substance P and associated neuropeptides (VIP and CGRP) may induce a rostral spread of nociception to the trigeminal nerve.[79] This was supported by the alleviation of a cluster headache attack by the administration of somatostatin, a substance P inhibitor.[80]

The trigeminovascular mechanisms discussed in the previous chapter dealing with migraine are also pertinent to cluster headache.[81] The cavernous sinus appears to be an important site in the etiology of cluster headache pain. It would also explain, neuroanatomically, the site of the cluster headache and the autonomic signs associated with the cluster headache attack.

We have discussed above the sympathetic nervous system changes in cluster headache. It is also felt that there are parasympathetic nervous system events which affect cluster headache. One suggestion was that the efferent impulses from the greater superficial petrosal nerves, which come from the parasympathetic nuclei in the hypothalamus, may induce the cluster headache.[82] Another author[83] noted that the excessive release of acetylcholine from parasympathetic nerve terminals could stimulate histamine release from mast cells, and this and other neurochemical pain mediators would stimulate nociceptors directly, leading to increased pain and the release of substance P, causing more pain, inflammation, and histamine release.

It would therefore appear that cluster headache periods are associated with changes in normal neurophysiology. These changes include dysfunction of some regions of the hypothalamus which induce chronobiological abnormalities with impaired sympathetic and parasympathetic activity. This in turn would cause decreases in the autoregulatory function in vasomotor regulation and chemoreceptor responses to hypoxemia. Sustained hypoxemia, secondary to diminished carotid body activity, could create the pathophysiological environment for the cluster attack. Pathways of the cluster headache may involve cranial nerves V, VII, IX, and X. These cranial nerve changes may induce, via neurotransmitter changes, hemodynamic changes in the arteries and veins which affect nociception and the associated signs and symptoms of the cluster headache.

Therapy

As for migraine headache, the therapy for cluster headache may be considered as being abortive or prophylactic, although the abortive agents work better, clinically, in episodic cluster patients. It is most beneficial, as patients may have more than one cluster headache a day, to utilize prophylactic treatment during an episodic cluster period and use the abortives for breakthrough headaches. This requires knowing the average length of a patient's cluster period and slowly weaning them off the prophylactic medications around the end of the cluster period.

One of the most useful abortives, in terms of success rates, is the use of 100% oxygen given at the rate of 7 liters per minute by facial mask. Most headaches will stop within 15 minutes. There is a clinical suspicion that over-utilization of oxygen may increase the frequency of cluster headaches. A major problem with the use of oxygen is that many cluster attacks will occur during the day when a patient is at work or at another activity, making the use of a small tank of oxygen useful, but problematic.

A rapidly acting form of ergotamine tartrate may be useful. This would include the sublingual tablet, intranasal sprays (DHE), and rectal suppositories. The absorption rate of oral forms of ergotamine is too slow to help patients with a cluster lasting 45 to 60 minutes.

In patients who experience a cluster headache routinely during the first REM stage of sleep, 90 to 120 minutes after they fall asleep, taking two ergotamine tablets immediately before going to sleep will enable the medication to be at a peak plasma level and typically abort the headache. It should be noted that migraine patients who take ergotamine too frequently will develop vascular rebound headaches. For some possibly metabolic reason, the cluster patient can take the ergot preparations daily and not develop rebound.

The use of intranasal Stadol is a good abortive, but caution must be taken to avoid rebound from this drug, even though it is a narcotic antagonist-agonist. This medication can have side effects ranging from burning in the sinuses to patients feeling "weird" and "hyper". Some patients may hallucinate after using the medication, so where and when the medication is used must be considered. Its addiction potential has been markedly underrated.

The use of sumatriptan subcutaneously is also very promising for aborting a cluster headache, although the cost of the medication may hinder some patients, and its use more than once a day may also be problematic. Another abortive medication is lidocaine in a 4% aqueous solution applied by a dropper or a pledget to the sphenopalatine ganglia. In the past, cocaine was utilized in this fashion and gave good relief for cluster headache, probably better than lidocaine, as cocaine is a sympathomimetic agent. Problems with possible addiction and legality clearly reduce the practicality of this approach. A problem with the use of intranasal lidocaine is that, for best results, the patient must lie down and position his head properly for the medication to reach the sphenopalatine ganglia, making this agent also problematic to use, depending on where patients are when they need the medication.

Prophylactic treatment is used for both episodic and chronic cluster. It is more difficult in chronic cluster patients, who may need to change their medications periodically. Also making it more difficult is the fact that most chronic cluster patients, as well as some episodic cluster patients, may need a combination of prophylactic medications to achieve relief. It is therefore incumbent upon the clinician to understand the various aspects of these drugs, alone and in combination with other medications.

Methysergide is useful for episodic cluster headache prophylaxis. It is given in divided doses of 4 to 10 mg a day and must be titrated to optimal effectiveness. It is also useful as a single therapy, at least initially, for cluster headache patients. It should not be used for repeated bouts of cluster, as tachyphylaxis may develop, making it ineffective. In some cases, the addition of a corticosteroid in these patients can restore the effectiveness of the drug. The use of methysergide should be limited to 5 to 6 months. The continuous use of the medication longer than 6 months can induce retroperitoneal fibrosis, as well as fibrotic changes in the lungs and heart valves. The medication should be tapered slowly and patients given at least a 1- to 2-month drug holiday before it is re-introduced. All patients should be given laboratory tests, chest X-rays, and intravenous pyelograms to rule out any end organ damage from prolonged or repeated use of the medication.

The use of ergotamine tartrate is an alternative to methysergide. It is given in low doses (.6 mg), alone or in a combination preparation such as Bellergal-S. It should be used twice daily. Patients should be re-evaluated monthly for side effects of the medication. They should be weaned off slowly, starting 2 to 3 weeks after their last cluster headache.

Lithium carbonate is an excellent prophylactic treatment for chronic cluster. It can also be used for the episodic cluster patient. The dosage is between 300 and 900 mg a day in divided doses. Blood levels should be monitored. It may be started as a single drug, but if efficacy is lost then a second drug can be added, such as verapamil. The drug action is not well understood, although it appears to work in the hypothalamus, possibly in the region of the supraoptic nucleus, as it may help by restoring chronobiological homeostasis. It does have serotonergic properties. Similar to the use of the ergots, cluster patients may take more lithium without the side effects seen in bipolar patients, such as shakiness, dizziness, and subjective cognitive changes.

Verapamil is also useful in both episodic and chronic cluster headache. It may be used in combination with other medications ... carefully! It takes about 2 weeks for the drug to be effective for episodic cluster, with an average dosage of 350 mg a day. The chronic cluster patient may take 4 to 5 weeks to show a response, at dosages averaging 572 mg a day, in divided dosages. Time-release formulations are useful. Another calcium channel blocker, nimodopine, is also useful at 120 mg a day.

Corticosteroids can also be used. In the episodic cluster patient, a 10-day burst treatment with prednisone, starting at 80 mg and weaning down to 0 over 10 days, is helpful. Some clinicians have used prednisone on a daily basis at 10 to 80 mg a day, the average being 40 mg. Responsiveness was good, although in some patients their headaches returned as the steroid was decreased. Low-dose ergotamine or lithium carbonate may be given concomitantly with the prednisone. In the chronic cluster patient, it may be possible to wean the prednisone after several days. Valproic acid, given at doses of 500 to 750 mg a day, may also be used alone or, carefully, in combination with ergotamine tartrate and possibly lithium for chronic cluster.

Histamine desensitization, using intravenous histamine infusions of 5.5 mg of histamine phosphate per 24 hours for 10 days may be useful in the treatment of intractable cluster headache. This is done in combination with H_1 and H_2 antagonists. This technique may be useful in chronic cluster patients who have lost their ability to respond to lithium carbonate or verapamil. After the intravenous treatment, responsiveness to these drugs may be restored. In general, this technique is not given a great deal of credence, for several historical reasons, particularly its unsuccessful overutilization for all types of headaches in the past. Also, there is a paucity of well-controlled studies. The use of oral agents — 200 mg a day of cimetidine, an H_2 antagonist, and 20 mg a day of chlorpheniramine, an H_1 antagonist, individually or together — has not been markedly successful in the treatment of cluster headaches.

There are several surgical procedures utilized for the totally conservatively untreatable chronic cluster patient. These procedures include sectioning the greater superficial petrosal nerve, which is no longer in favor; section of the nervus intermedius, which can lead to sterile inflammatory reactions secondary to parasympathetic discharges; destruction of the sphenopalatine ganglion, which has provided short duration and/or incomplete relief and is rarely performed; and percutaneous radiofrequency gasserian ganglion lesioning, which is the preferred technique. Radiofrequency thermocoagulation of the gasserian ganglion leads to good relief of trigeminal neuralgia. The usefulness of this procedure has been validated in cluster headache. It produces abolition of the corneal reflex ipsilaterally, which promises at least a 66% chance of pain relief, which will last until the corneal reflex recovers, typically over several years. Some of these patients do experience painless attacks of ptosis, tearing, and rhinorrhea. Local anesthetic blocks should be done first to evaluate the patient for the more invasive procedure. Retrogasserian injection of glycerol has also been useful. With this procedure, pain relief correlated with the degree of corneal sensory loss. Trigeminal root sectioning in the posterior fossa has been used as a last resort in treatment-resistant patients. Aside from corneal anesthesia, there is also an unpredictable risk of anesthesia dolorosa, or painful numbness. These risks may be considered acceptable for the treatment-resistant sufferers of intractable chronic cluster headache.

Chronic paroxysmal hemicrania

Chronic paroxysmal hemicrania (CPH) is a form of cluster headache first described in 1974. The attacks are much shorter (3 to 5 minutes) than cluster headache, but they occur from 4 to 38 times a day. The pain is typically in the same areas as cluster headache. The main differentiation is that CPH is exquisitely sensitive to indomethacin and *not* responsive to anticluster medications.

Indomethacin is given in doses of 25 to 50 mg three times a day. In some patients, the time-release form (given every 12 hours) may be used. Side effects include gastrointestinal problems, as well as bruising. Liver functions as well as CBC should be monitored at least every 2 to 3 months after an initial 1-month check.

Case study
RC is a 42-year-old righthanded Caucasian female first seen 5 years ago with a history of "migraine" which was seasonal, by history, and went back for 7 years. The unilateral headache pain was excruciating, she stated. The headaches lasted between 1 and 2 hours and were associated with ipsilateral tearing, nasal discharge, and redness of the eye. She had been taking both codeine and acetaminophen, as well butalbatal and aspirin, alone and together, and they did not help her pain.

She explained that the headaches were behind her left eye and had always been there. She became agitated when she had a headache and was unable to stay still. She had two to three headaches a day, one in the morning an hour after she awakened, one at 3:00 p.m., and one after she fell asleep. They were, to quote her, "as regular as clock work." She experienced these headaches for three or four months at a time, twice a year. The pain was terrible, excruciating, and felt like "something hot trying to push my eye out of my head." She also described another type of headache which was band-like around her head, aching in nature, and "relatively mild" in comparison to the other headaches. Her family physician and consulting neurologist had tried her on propranolol with no effect. She was at her wits end and wanted to know what was going on.

Examination revealed a minimal degree of ptosis on the left, but she was otherwise normal. Her diagnoses were episodic cluster headache and analgesic rebound headache. She was weaned off of the analgesics, slowly, particularly since she had been on the barbiturate for over 3 years. Simultaneously, she was started on lithium carbonate, 300 mg three times a day. Blood work, including liver and renal functions, was taken before she started the lithium as a baseline. The same lab tests, including lithium levels, were taken every month for 3 months, then once every 3 months. She was also given oxygen as an abortive treatment. As she did not work, she did well with one large tank in her bedroom.

Her headaches resolved within 3 weeks. After 3 months, she was taken off of the lithium slowly and was headache free for 5 months before the cluster headaches resumed. She was again placed on the lithium and did well. She was weaned off in 4 months, and had a 3-month remission period. Over the next 2 years, the same pattern repeated itself. Of note was the shorter duration of her remission periods.

After three years, she had not had a remission for over a year, and her diagnosis was changed to chronic cluster. Her lithium had been increased to four a day, and she remained in the mid-therapeutic range. Then she began again to have breakthrough headaches, so time-release verapamil (240 mg twice a day) was added. She continued to use the oxygen for headache breakthrough. She also started taking two tablets of 2-mg ergotamine tartrate before bed, which stopped the nocturnal headaches.

Five months later she began to complain of a different type of headache, as well as problems sleeping. Her cluster headaches were under good control. History showed her to be under a great deal of familial stress, including the death of a relative. Examination showed a cervical myofascial pain syndrome and reduced cervical range of motion. She was treated with a short course of physical therapy, as well as 20 mg of amitriptyline at night. She continued on lithium carbonate (300 mg four times a day), time-release verapamil (240 mg twice a day), and two ergotamine tartrate tablets at night.

The tension-type headache problem was relieved. Over the course of the next year, we spent time changing her medication dosages when she would develop breakthrough headaches for more than a week at a time. Her headaches remained under good control until a year and a half ago, when she began to complain of a new type of headache. This headache had been present for 3 weeks and was described as a sharp, stabbing, almost electrical type of pain that lasted for 3 to 5 minutes. It occurred 20 to 30 times a day and was located between her left temple and her left eye. Neurological examination was unchanged. She was started on indomethacin, one 75-mg, sustained-release tablet in the morning. The next day her new headache type was gone. Chronic paroxysmal hemicrania was added to her diagnosis list.

She developed some gastric discomfort but there were no complaints of black or tarry stools. Her CBC was normal. We cut the amount of indomethacin and divided the dosages. Her CPH returned. We increased the medication again, still to be taken with food. A week later, we tried to wean down the lithium, but her cluster headaches returned. The lithium carbonate was again increased to four a day. Then we decreased her verapamil to one a day. She remained controlled for 2 weeks, then the clusters returned, so the verapamil was increased to twice a day.

Over the next few months, without medical supervision, she adjusted her own indomethacin dose. Decreasing it always brought a return of CPH. For the next 6 months, she was stable and both cluster and CPH were under good control. The CPH then broke through again, necessitating an increase of her dosage to one 75-mg indomethacin tablet every 12 hours. This brought her CPH back under control.

Two months later she developed severe stomach pain and was sent to a gastroenterologist, who performed endoscopy. She was found to have a duodenal ulcer. By default, therefore, we were forced to stop the indomethacin. Unfortunately, the CPH returned within days. The pain was so great that the patient re-started her indomethacin without medical advice. She was seen again 2 weeks later, complaining of shortness of breath. She was pale and shaky. CBC showed a marked drop in her hematocrit and hemoglobin. She was transported from the office to the hospital, where her family physician decided not to transfuse her, but instead observed her in the hospital off of the indomethacin. Her blood work showed slow, gradual improvement and she was sent home after 5 days.

She saw me the next day and stated she was feeling suicidal because of the return of the CPH, for which she had been given Demerol shots around the clock in the hospital. The dilemma was, of course, that CPH is only sensitive to indomethacin, which was contraindicated because of her ulcer and gastrointestinal bleeding. The patient and I had a phone conference with her family physician. We were able to compromise, with

> the patient being allowed to restart her indomethacin if she would have a CBC done weekly at her family physician's office. She agreed.
>
> Since that time, she has remained in good control of both her cluster headache and the CPH. On occasion she has had some bleeding, but her physician places her under closer control, as do we. She is an intelligent woman who understands the ramifications of both her headache problems and the medication management problems. Her treatment continues, with weekly to monthly "fine tuning" of her medication. She remains headache free, with minimal cluster or CPH break-through.

Such medication management issues demonstrate the need for art, as well as science, in the treatment of headache. The most interesting aspect of this case is that the patient is a female cluster headache sufferer who developed chronic paroxysmal hemicrania. She also had an interval during which she developed tension-type headaches.

Of my two favorite medical sayings, one seems very appropriate here: "Even a schizophrenic can get hit by a truck." Or, stated differently, "A patient with lice can still have fleas." Bottom line, it is necessary to re-evaluate your patients continually if there are changes in their headaches. Do not lock yourself into a single, unchangeable diagnosis with any patient. To do so can be fatal. Literally.

Some years ago I was called to see a patient with a long history of low back pain. For over 10 years, she would experience an exacerbation of her pain, at which time her physician would hospitalize her for about a week and give her physical therapy, traction, and medications which gave her significant help. Then she would be discharged. I was called to see her after she was in the hospital for almost 2 weeks. None of the medications or therapy which, in the past, had been so helpful appeared to be working. When I went into the nurses' station to get her chart, the nurse chuckled and commented about the "back pain patient in room XXX." I examined her, and the bottom line is this. She *was* the back pain patient in room XXX, and she had been thought of that way for so long that nobody bothered to thoroughly re-examine her. I found a pancreatic tumor. She died within 2 months.

It is dangerous to let your thinking about a headache patient be "fixed" on one diagnosis. Whenever there is a change in a patient's report of intensity, duration, or frequency of headache, you should check it out. Again, don't get locked into one way of thinking.

Another patient had a long history of migraine. The patient was a 27-year-old male, and his headaches were under good control. One evening he called the office complaining of a severe headache that was "sort of like my bad migraines." He was very sorry to call, he explained, as he thought it was just one of his typical migraines. Questioning revealed that he had been playing football several hours earlier, and his headache began while he was playing.

He was asked to meet me in the hospital emergency room. Examination showed some meningeal signs, and a CAT scan revealed a subarachnoid hemorrhage. Angiography showed some vascular spasm. He was admitted to the hospital and had a neurosurgical consult. The neurosurgeon wanted to observe the patient. We did, the bleeding resolved, and the patient was given the diagnosis of idiopathic subarachnoid hemorrhage. He was discharged in a week. There has been no recurrence.

I was really glad that he called. Needless to say, so was he. So, never identify the patient by their headache type. It may change when you least expect it.

The next chapter deals with the most common type of headache, acute and chronic tension-type headache. We will have to expand our knowledge base again to "get it". So, lets move on!

chapter five

Tension-type headache: clinical and pathophysiological aspects

One of the simplest and yet most complex headache problems is that of tension-type headache. It is the most common headache problem seen, both alone and in conjunction with other types of headache.

The name itself — tension-type headache — is indicative of the uncertain etiology of this entity. Is it physical, emotional, or a combination of both? It is more appropriate, however, to determine the various aspects of the disorder by looking at the underlying central nervous system pathophysiology in regard to the physical and emotional aspects of this headache entity.

Tension-type headache is differentiated into two forms, episodic and chronic. According to the Headache Classification Committee of the IHS,[12] The basic differentiating qualification is that the episodic form occurs less than 15 times a month, while the chronic form occurs 15 or more days a month. But, oh, there is much more, as you shall see.

Questions to be answered include one as to whether the chronic (or daily) tension-type headache is an extension of migraine — that is, do patients with episodic migraine "transform" that type of headache into chronic daily tension-type headache? This author does not believe this to be the case. Furthermore, the evidence is extensive to the contrary.

Also, we must here differentiate between what is being called chronic or daily headache and chronic and daily tension-type headache. The former indicates daily headache of mixed type, as you will see. The latter is only one type of headache which may be part of the former. Well, since this type of straightforward talk always confuses me even further, let us move on to the facts themselves.

As complex as many may consider migraine and cluster headache, it is felt by the author that tension-type headache is even more complex, as well as being more difficult in its chronic form to diagnose and treat. But, you can make your own mind up about that.

Clinical aspects

The new classification system[12] describes the diagnostic criteria of episodic tension-type headache as being recurrent headache occurring fewer than 15 days a month and lasting from 30 minutes to 7 days. At least two of four pain characteristics are present: pain with a pressing/tightening (non-pulsating) quality; pain which is mild to moderate in intensity and may inhibit, but not prohibit, activities; pain which is always bilateral; and pain which is not aggravated by walking stairs or doing other routine physical activity. Finally, the new classification system states that both of the following are true: (1) there is no nausea or vomiting, but anorexia may occur, and (2) photophobia and phonophobia are absent, or one but not the other is present. Of course, organic disorders have been ruled out by the initial examination or by imaging studies; if disease is present, the headaches should not have started in a close temporal relationship to the disorder. On a clinical basis, it appears that several important clinical aspects were not taken into consideration when these criteria were drawn up, as you will see.

The diagnosis of episodic tension-type headache is typically a diagnosis of exclusion. If it is not migraine or cluster headache, or it is not another primary headache disorder, and there is no organic causation, it is an episodic tension-type headache.

The pain is typically aching or pressure-like, frequently described as being "like a vice around my head." Other descriptions include a tight band around the head, or "like wearing a tight bathing cap over my head." The pain is usually bilateral, but it may be unilateral. It may include some or all of these areas: occipito-nuchal, bifrontal, bitemporal, suboccipital, at the vertex of the head, or extending into the neck and shoulders.

The intensity of the pain may wax and wane. The episodic headache may occur during times of stress or in anticipation of a stressful event. It frequently may occur towards the end of the work day. The emotional/psychological aspects of this type of headache have been, in the past, used as diagnostic excuses, as they may or may not be present, in spite of the pejorative past diagnosis of "tension headache".

There is a female predominance, although it is not as great as in migraine. Episodic tension-type headache may begin in adolescence and in young adults. Children also may have the problem. Typically, the headaches are noted to begin in patients between 20 and 40 years of age.

Unlike migraine patients, episodic tension-type headache patients may carry on with their activities, although most take some form of analgesic. Many clinicians like to see evidence of emotional difficulties such as anxiety and tension, and they often describe the patients as sitting rigidly on the edge of their seats, rather than being relaxed. Forgotten is the fear many patients have of physicians and particularly of finding out their headaches are secondary to a brain tumor or something equally horrendous.

Few physicians adequately look for evidence of excessive or sustained muscle contraction, except for palpating the pericranial muscles. They equate lack of muscle spasm or pain to a psychogenic cause for the headaches. Muscle exhaustion (secondary to chronic spasm eliminating the continued metabolic ability to maintain the spasm) is a foreign concept, on occasion.

This author also feels that it is strange that the diagnostic criteria place oromandibular dysfunction under the category of tension-type headache. Also under this classification are temporomandibular joint dysfunction (TMJ), myofascial pain dysfunction (MPD), and craniomandibular dysfunction. It seems to this author, as well as to other specialists, that MPD and TMJ are separate entities which may be associated with tension-type headache.

The International Headache Society places tenderness as a distinct subheading, while stating that oromandibular dysfunction must have three of six features: TMJ noise on jaw movement, limited or jerky jaw movements, pain on jaw function, locking of jaw on opening, clenching or grinding of teeth, or other parafunctions of the tongue, lips, or cheek (biting or pressing). Other clinicians, including the author (who performed a study to investigate the question of TMJ crepitus or noise), have found that there is no true clinical relationship between crepitus and TMJ pain or dysfunction.

The clinical aspects of TMJ dysfunction include limitations of jaw opening (15 or 16 mm or less), jaw deviation to one side when the mouth is opened, and crepitus. Typically, there is also pain or tenderness in the area of the TMJ or the muscles of mastication. Imaging studies should be positive for disc displacement or ligamentous difficulties. In point of clinical fact, the vast majority of patients seen with the diagnosis of TMJ, even after diagnosis and treatment by our colleagues in dentistry, have as their primary problem tenderness or pain (with or without palpable spasm) of the muscles of mastication. This diagnosis is correct more than 98% of the time, and conservative physical therapy or even a trigger point injection into the lateral pterygoid muscle will stop the pain, without appliances or dental work.

Patients with episodic tension-type headache may also have migraine, even as patients with lice can have fleas. Some patients have "mixed vascular and episodic tension-type headaches". It is from "features" such as this that the idea of migraine headache "transforming" to tension-type or chronic daily headaches arose, although this author does not agree with this supposition.

As defined above, chronic tension-type headache occurs 15 or more days a month for at least 6 months.[12] This is the most common diagnosis seen in headache specialty clinics, either alone or as one of the various diagnoses in a "combination headache" patient.

These patients have headache daily or every other day. They note that their headaches are there when they awaken and remain until they go to sleep. The pain varies in intensity, typically downward, for several hours after analgesics are taken. Some of these patients indicate that the "true" headache lasts for hours a day, but there is also a constant nagging ache which is amenable to distraction.

Chronic tension-type headaches have been subdivided into two types: those with associated pericranial muscle spasm or pain and those without. The latter group was once termed, inappropriately, "chronic psychogenic headache".

Various authorities, but not all by any means, feel that chronic tension-type headache occurs either from "transformation" from episodic migraine or from rebound headache from various types of medication. They feel that in a minority of cases chronic tension-type headache will evolve from episodic tension-type headache, as well as occur *de novo*, or by itself. It is only after one is fully aquainted with the pathophysiology that one should make such statements.

Patients with chronic tension-type headache may have aspects of depression as well as anxiety. Many clinicians look at this as a "chicken and egg" problem of which came first. Again, looking at the neurochemistry of chronic tension-type headache will help answer that question.

The differential diagnosis is again one of exclusion. If it is not migraine or cluster or CPH, and there is no organic cause of headache, then it must be tension-type, and if it occurs more than 15 days a month, then it is chronic tension-type headache. Some clinicians do look at the question of cervicogenic headache, but this diagnosis is dismissed by the majority of American physicians. Headache caused by organic diseases of the head and neck, as well as by systemic diseases, often begins with intermittent episodic headaches and evolves into chronic daily headache as the underlying disease process progresses. So, without further ado, let us move into an explanation of some of the proposed mechanisms of this problem.

Pathophysiology of tension-type headache

The diagnostic criteria for acute and chronic tension-type headache have been noted above. You should note that these criteria are not exact nor do they encompass all clinical aspects of acute or chronic tension-type headache (A/CTTHA). Pathological changes in the musculoskeletal system may initiate, modulate, or perpetuate A/CTTHA. Episodic and chronic tension-type headache are, at least at first, a muscle-induced pain syndrome which is frequently associated with the myofascial pain syndrome and/or fibromyalgia.[84]

The central nervous system controls muscle tone via systems including gamma efferent neurons in the anterior horn cells of the spinal cord, which act on the alpha motor neurons supplying muscle spindles. Renshaw cells, probably via the inhibitory neurotransmitter gamma aminobutyric acid (GABA), influence this synaptic system. There is also supraspinal control mediated by the cortical, subcortical, and limbic afferent and efferent systems. Physiological and emotional inputs interact in the maintenance or flux of established muscle tone. Adverse influences from both localized or regional myofascial nociception, with or without limbic (affective) stimulation, may produce significant muscle spasm which, if prolonged, becomes tonic with the additional aspects of increased anxiety or a maintained muscle contraction-pain cycle.[85,86] This helps to differentiate acute vs. chronic tension-type headache, to a degree.

Tonic or continued muscle contraction may induce hypoxia via compression of small blood vessels. Ischemia, the accumulation of pain-producing metabolites (bradykinin, lactic acid, serotonin, prostoglandins, etc.), may increase and potentiate muscle pain and reactive spasm. These nociception-enhancing chemicals may stimulate central mechanisms which, through continued stimulation, may induce continued reactive muscle contraction and maintenance of the myogenic nociceptive cycle.[87–89]

Some researchers have confirmed a causal relationship between muscle spasm and headache,[90–92] while others have felt that associated muscle spasm is an epiphenomenon, not the cause of headache[93–98] but a reflexive response rather than an etiological mechanism. Other authors have indicated that muscle activity/spasm may be more pronounced in migraine than in tension-type/muscle contraction headaches.[99,100]

A major problem with this research, in which information was obtained by electromyographic (EMG) studies, was that the authors evaluated different groups of muscles in different types of patients, many of whom had poorly defined diagnoses.[91,99,101,102] Other authors defined chronic tension-type headache as an entity with or without associated pericranial muscle disorder.[103] The concept of muscle fatigue was not taken into consideration; metabolically spent muscles may become relatively flaccid, losing aspects of increased tone or spasm.

Langemark and Olesen[104] found that there was a positive correlation between pericranial muscle tenderness and headache intensity, and the former was felt to be the source of nociception. In another study,[105] Langemark et al. found that pressure pain thresholds in patients with chronic tension-type headache were highly dependent on myofascial factors. This study indicated that the generally lower pain thresholds in the chronic tension-type headache patients suggested a dysmodulation of central nociception. A lower pain threshold in chronic tension-type headache patients, as compared to normal volunteers, was also noted by Borgeat et al.[106]

Drummond,[107] who measured scalp muscle tenderness and sensitivity to pain in both migraine and tension-type headache patients, felt that the pathophysiology of tension-type headache may involve a diffuse disruption of central pain-modulating mechanisms. Lower pain thresholds were also found in patients diagnosed with myofascial pain syndromes, including lower back pain.[108,109]

The chronic tension-type headache patients frequently have a stereotypic posture, with their shoulders raised and their heads held in forward flexion. This tightly held posture, or muscular splinting, is effective in preventing unconscious head movement which may induce increased pain. The continued splinting, by maintaining tonic muscle contraction, also works to increase myogenic nociception and perpetuate the cycle.

The pericranial muscles are innervated by sensory fibers in nerves from the second or third cervical roots and in the trigeminal nerve.[110] The functions of these muscles contribute to the maintenance of posture and the stabilization of the head, as well as the withdrawal and protection of the head. These factors certainly contribute to their role in the myofascial aspects of chronic tension-type headache.

Muscle fatigue, both metabolic and neurochemical in nature, which may follow prolonged or tonic muscle spasm, may also be secondary to "sympatheticopenia", or the depletion of epinephrine and norepinephrine, the peripheral sympathetic transmitters.[111] The muscle spindle is directly affected by the sympathetic nervous system via neurotransmitters, particularly norepinephrine (NEP). Prolonged and sustained peripheral sympathetic activity may lead to depletion of NEP at the synaptic receptors. Continued afferent sympathetic input from myogenic nociception, at least in part from buildup through ischemia of nociceptive metabolites, may result in sympatheticopenia.[111,112]

Also correlated positively with pericranial muscle tenderness is tenderness of the cervical, thoracic, and lumbar paravertebral muscles.[113] Murphy and Lehrer[114] indicated that contraction of shoulder and cervical muscles as well as emotional arousal contribute to tension-type headache.

Three mechanisms of muscle pain are thought to be relevant to acute, but more often to chronic, tension-type headache, in that myogenic nociception may be induced by: (1) low-grade inflammation associated with the release of algetic, or pain-inducing substances, rather than signs of acute inflammation, (2) short- or long-lasting relative ischemia, and (3) tearing of ligaments and tendons secondary to abnormal, sustained muscle tension.[110]

Myofascial pain syndrome (MPS)

Travell and Rinzler[115] identified the contribution of musculoskeletal factors in the etiology of acute and chronic tension-type headache. They demonstrated that there are consistent patterns of referred pain from trigger points within specific muscles and defined perpetuating factors that convert acute myofascial pain into a chronic pain syndrome.[116]

The myofascial pain syndrome is a localized or regional pain problem associated with small zones of hypersensitivity within skeletal muscle called trigger points. With palpation of these points, pain is referred to adjacent or even distant sites. Trigger points in the head, neck, and upper back may elicit headache, as well as tinnitus, vertigo, and lacrimation, all features noted in patients with chronic tension-type headache.[117] (See Figures 1 through 8.)

Trigger points may be active, with consistently reproducible pain on palpation, or latent, with no clinically associated complaints of pain but with

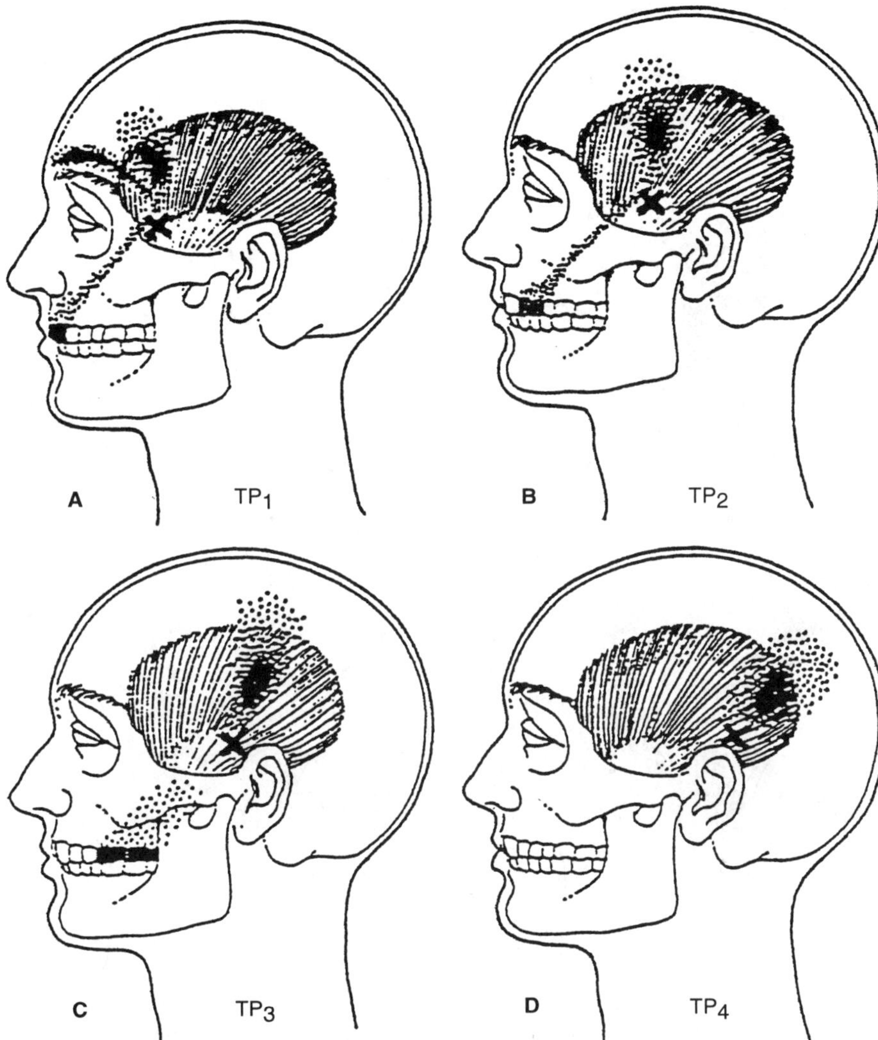

Figure 1 Referred pain patterns from trigger points (×) in the left temporalis muscle. Dark areas show essential zones; spillover zones are stippled. **(A)** Anterior "spokes" of pain arising from the anterior fibers — trigger point 1 region. **(B)** and **(C)** Middle spokes — trigger point 2 and 3 regions. **(D)** Posterior supra-auricular spoke — trigger point 4 region. (From Jay, G.W., in *Treating the Headache Patient,* Cady, R.K. and Fox, A.W. (Eds.) Marcel Dekker, New York, 1995, pp. 211–233. With permission.)

associated muscle dysfunction. Trigger points may shift between active and latent states. Clinically, continuous myogenic nociception from active trigger points appears to be a prime instigator of the central neurochemical nociceptive dysmodulation found in patients with chronic tension-type headache.

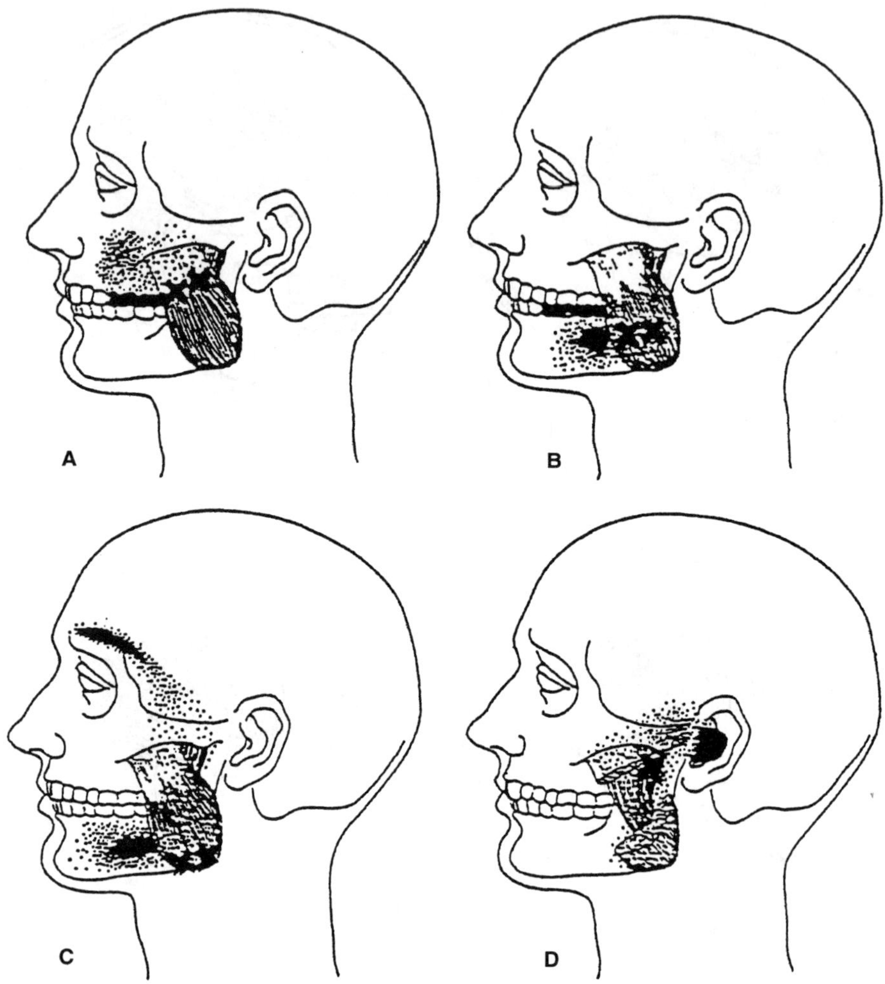

Figure 2 Each × indicates a trigger point in various parts of the masseter muscle. Dark areas show essential zones; spillover zones are stippled. **(A)** Superficial layer, upper portion. **(B)** Superficial layer, mid-belly. **(C)** Superficial layer, lower portion. **(D)** Deep layer, upper part — just below the temporomandibular joint. (From Jay, G.W., in *Treating the Headache Patient*, Cady, R.K. and Fox, A.W. (Eds.) Marcel Dekker, New York, 1995, pp. 211–233. With permission.)

Increased stiffness, weakness, and fatigue and a decreased range of motion may be found in muscles in which trigger points are found. These muscles may be shortened, with increased pain perceived on stretching. Patients may protect these muscles by adapting poor posture with sustained contraction (see above).[110,118] The resulting muscular restrictions may perpetuate existing trigger points and aid in the development of others.

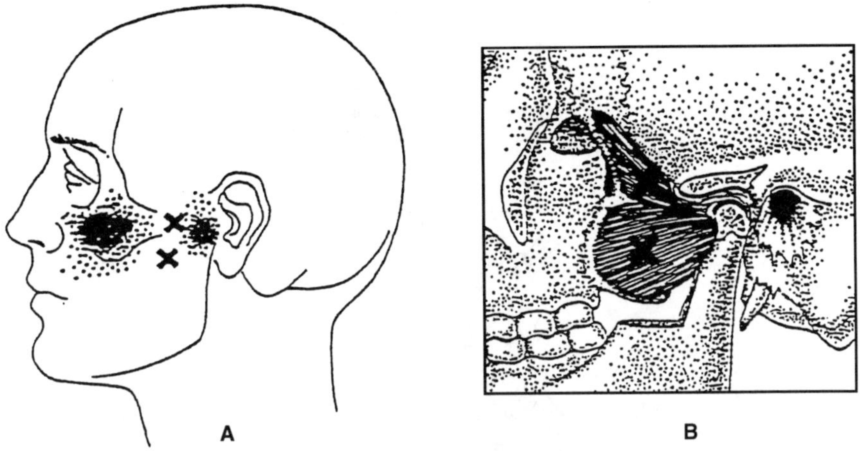

Figure 3 Referred pain pattern **(A)** of trigger points (×) in the left lateral pterygoid muscle **(B)**. Note the similarity to temporomandibular disorder. (From Jay, G.W., in *Treating the Headache Patient*, Cady, R.K. and Fox, A.W. (Eds.) Marcel Dekker, New York, 1995, pp. 211–233. With permission.)

Fricton et. al.[119] noted that a large percentage of patients suffering from MPS of the head and neck were found to have significant postural problems, with forward head tilt and rounded shoulders, as well as poor standing and sitting posture, all findings frequently seen in chronic tension-type headache

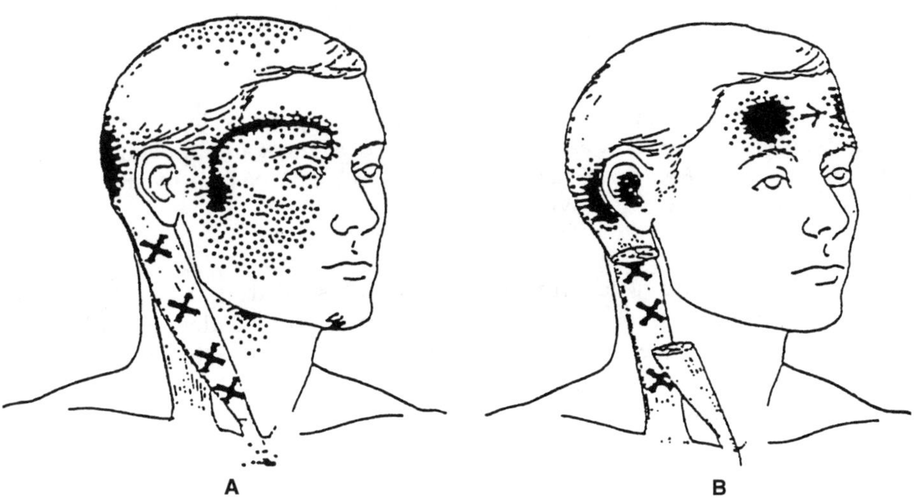

Figure 4 Referred pain patterns with location of corresponding trigger points (×) in the right sternocleidomastoid muscle. Dark areas show essential zones; spillover zones are stippled. **(A)** The sternal (superficial) division. **(B)** The clavicular (deep) dividion. (From Jay, G.W., in *Treating the Headache Patient*, Cady, R.K. and Fox, A.W. (Eds.) Marcel Dekker, New York, 1995, pp. 211–233. With permission.)

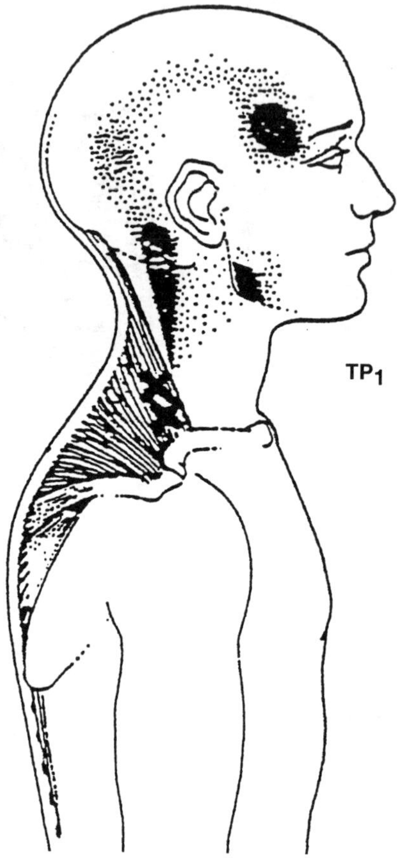

Figure 5 Referred pain pattern and location of trigger point (×) in the upper trapezius muscle. Dark areas show essential zones; spillover zones are stippled. (From Jay, G.W., in *Treating the Headache Patient,* Cady, R.K. and Fox, A.W. (Eds.) Marcel Dekker, New York, 1995, pp. 211–233. With permission.)

patients. MPS of the head and neck, via myofascial trigger point referred pain, may mimic other conditions, including migraine headache, TMJ disorders, sinusitis, and cervical neuralgias, as well as various otological problems including tinnitus, vertigo, ear pain, and dizziness.[118]

The onset of an acute, single-muscle MPS may be associated with trauma, such as a slip and fall, an acceleration/deceleration injury, or even a direct blow. It may also come on insidiously — for example, in patients who work multiple hours typing or at the computer. The MPS, in many patients, may show a spontaneous regression to a latent status, with continued muscular dysfunction, but with significant diminution of the initial pain complaints. In other patients, the MPS may "metastasize" and involve associated musculature, becoming regional, or even involving multiple muscular regions.

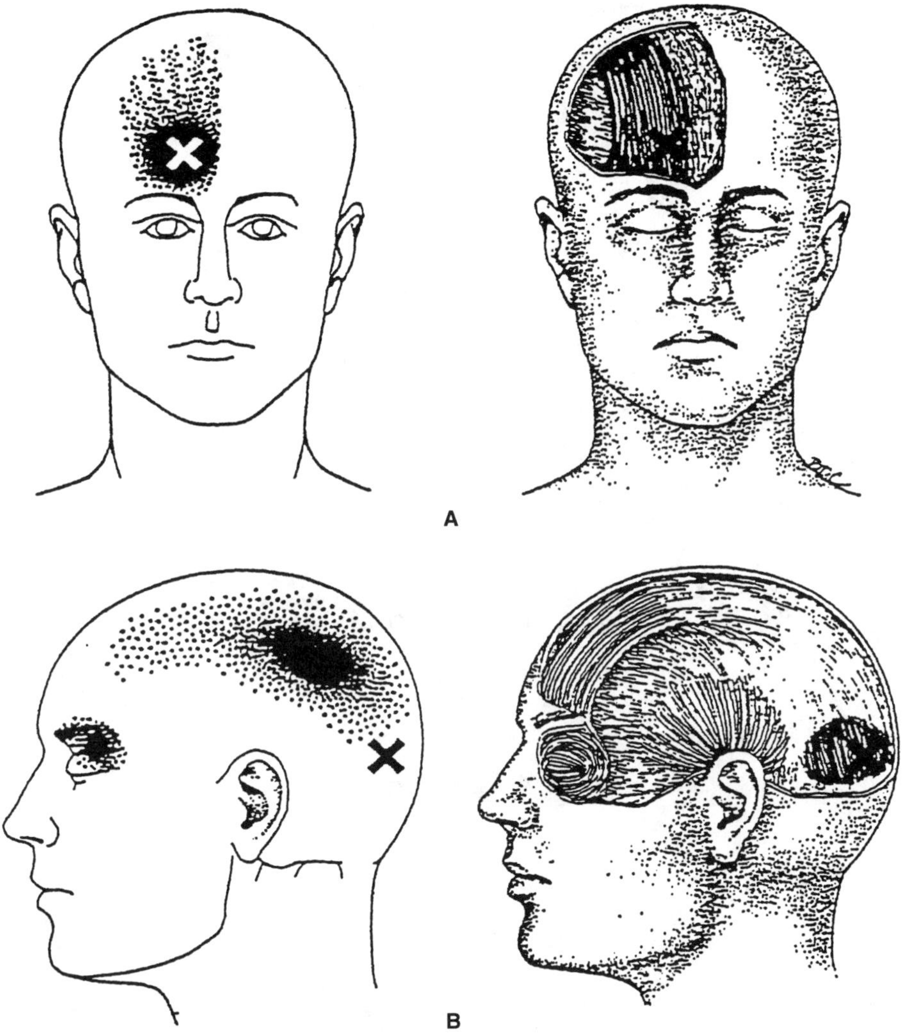

Figure 6 Pain patterns (shaded areas) referred from trigger points (×) in the occipitofrontalis muscle, commonly associated with unilateral, supraorbital, or ocular headache. **(A)** Right frontalis belly. **(B)** Left occipitalis belly. (From Jay, G.W., in *Treating the Headache Patient,* Cady, R.K. and Fox, A.W. (Eds.) Marcel Dekker, New York, 1995, pp. 211–233. With permission.)

Other clinical aspects

The exact role of emotional problems such as stress, anxiety, and depression is questionable, and the literature is equivocal. Either way, most researchers agree that emotional/psychological factors may be important in the maintenance, if not the genesis, of tension-type headaches.

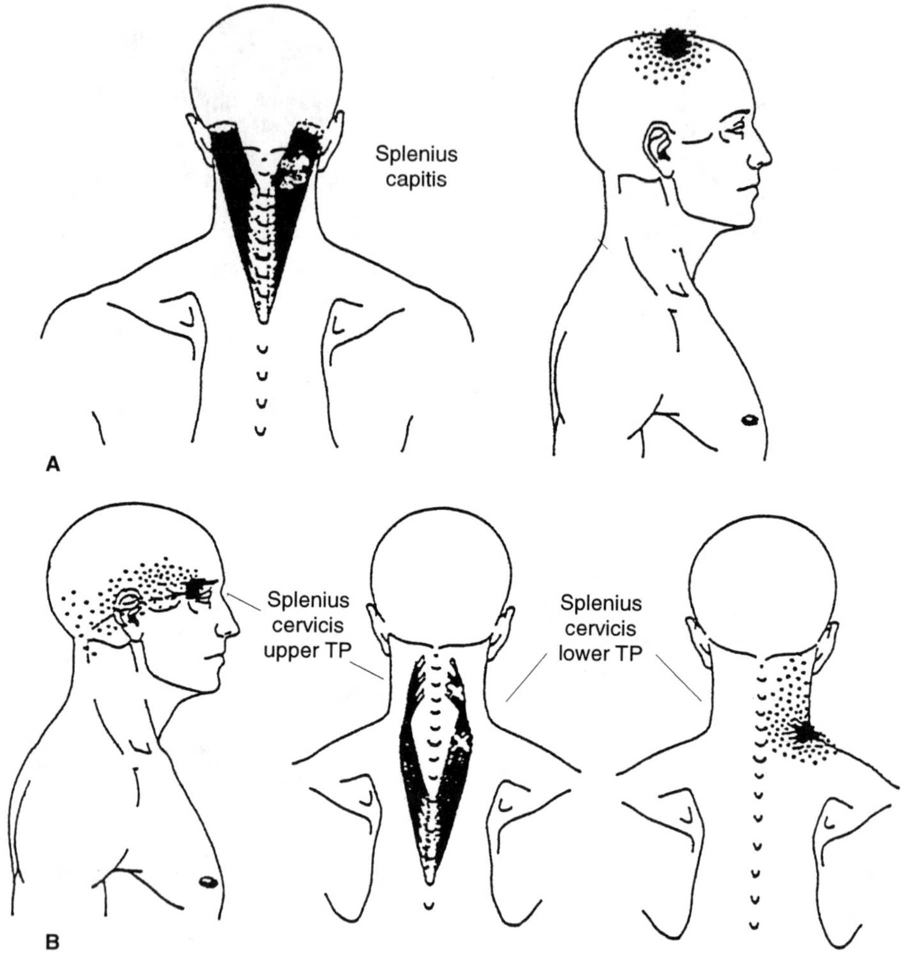

Figure 7 Trigger points (×) and referred pain patterns (shaded areas) for the right splenius capitis and splenius cervicis muscles. **(A)** The splenius capitis trigger point, which overlies the occipital triangle. **(B)** (Left) The upper splenius cervicis trigger point (TP) refers pain to the orbit. The dashed arrow represents the pain shooting from the inside of the head to the back of the eye. (Right) Another site of pain referral. (From Jay, G.W., in *Treating the Headache Patient,* Cady, R.K. and Fox, A.W. (Eds.) Marcel Dekker, New York, 1995, pp. 211–233. With permission.)

Depression has been linked to the initiation of tension-type headaches by some,[86,119] while others remain uncertain.[120] One difficulty revealed in the literature is the fact that determinations of depression, anxiety, and stress occur in patients with chronic tension-type headache. Without premorbid psychological analyses, it is obviously difficult to state with certainty whether these patients were depressed or anxious prior to the onset of their headache

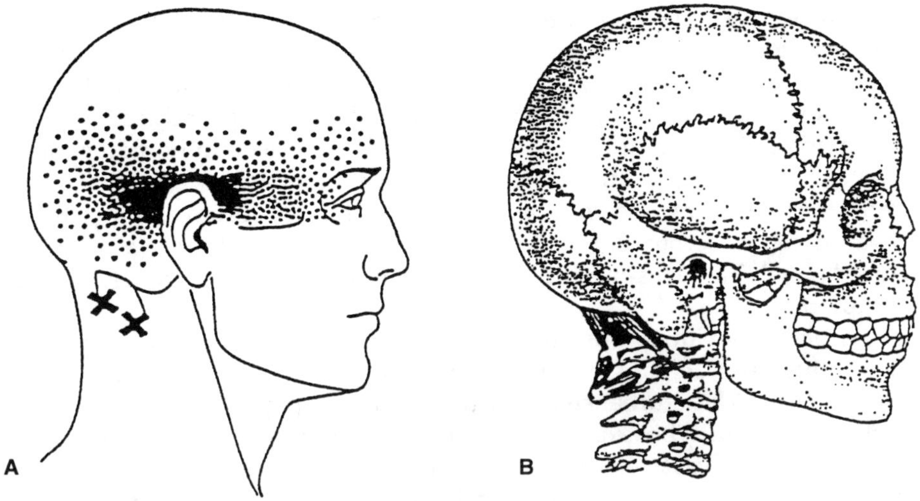

Figure 8 **(A)** Referred pain pattern (shaded area) of trigger points (×) in the right suboccipital muscles **(B)**. (From Jay, G.W., in *Treating the Headache Patient,* Cady, R.K. and Fox, A.W. (Eds.) Marcel Dekker, New York, 1995, pp. 211–233. With permission.)

problems. It is therefore possible that the neurochemical changes associated with chronic tension-type headache, such as a possible or probable central serotonergic dysfunction, initiate depression as a response to these pain-induced neurochemical changes.

Some authors have noted that the "conversion V" found in the hypochondriasis, depression, and hysteria scales of the Minnesota Multiphasic Personality Inventory (MMPI) is a marker for the tension-type headache patient, although similar responses are found in chronic non-headache pain patients.[121–123]

Associated sleep disorders

There appears to be an important relationship between sleep, headache, and the muscle-pain syndromes. Central biogenic amines, particularly serotonin and norepinephrine, are important to sleep physiology as well as to the central pain-modulating systems. Human and animal research indicates that central serotonin metabolism plays a role in pain modulation, affective states, and the regulation of non-REM sleep.[124]

A high incidence of sleep disturbance has been noted in chronic tension-type headache patients.[125] Different sleep disorders may be associated with different headache entities. Migraine has been found to occur in association with REM sleep, as well as excessive stage 3, 4, and REM sleep.[126] Chronic tension-type headache has been found to be associated with frequent awakenings and decreased slow-wave sleep, as well as an alpha-wave intrusion into stage 4 sleep.[127] The latter sleep changes are similar to those seen in fibromyalgia.

Moldofsky et al.[128] reported a disturbance in stage 4 sleep as the first laboratory-based abnormality found in fibromyalgia. They induced a similar alpha non-REM pattern of alpha intrusion in delta sleep in normal subjects by stage 4 sleep deprivation. Their subjects developed musculoskeletal pain and affective changes comparable to those seen in fibromyalgia patients. Small doses of serotonergic tricyclic antidepressant medications which reduced the alpha intrusions into stage 4 sleep were utilized to ameliorate the symptoms.

Alpha-wave intrusions into deep sleep have also been found in patients with other chronic pain syndromes, including rheumatoid arthritis.[129] The alpha non-REM disturbance has also been seen in asymptomatic people, as well as in those who experience severe emotional stress, such as combat veterans.[124] In the latter group, the veterans with this sleep disorder also complained of chronic headaches, diffuse pain, and emotional distress.

Sleep disturbance is associated with increased pain severity. As noted above, chronic headache patients seem to have a higher incidence of sleep abnormalities than do normal, pain-free subjects. Etiological aspects of chronic headache may be linked to sleep abnormalities as an initiating element or as a result of the underlying pathologically dysmodulated neurochemical factors inducing a sleep disorder.

Other possible associated factors

There are two possible mechanical etiologies of chronic tension-type headache. The first, cervical spondylosis, is defined as a degenerative disease affecting intervertebral discs and apophyseal joints of the cervical spine. While several authors note a possible correlation between cervical spondylosis and tension-type headache,[85,86,96] others conclude the contrary,[130] suggesting that the basis of existing headache is secondary to muscle contraction and/or central neurochemical dysmodulation.

The dental literature has been most active in reporting a possible correlation between TMJ dysfunction and tension-type headache (see above).[131,132] The relationship appears to depend mainly on tenderness of the masticatory muscles, which may have other etiologies and induce TMJ dysfunction, when it exists, on a secondary basis.[113,133,134]

Fibromyalgia

Fibromyalgia is a systemic disorder clinically associated with a generalized increase in tenderness in susceptible areas over the entire body. These specific tender points may induce a specific vulnerability to the central nociceptive pathways, much like myofascial trigger points.[134,135] Patients with fibromyalgia are typically women between the ages of 30 and 50, with complaints of generalized pain with bilateral, symmetric tenderness for at least 3 months. On physical examination, at least 11 of 18 symmetric tender points must be found to confirm the diagnosis.[136,137] The most common complaints found in these patients include morning stiffness, fatigue, chronic tension-type headaches, sleep disturbances, and irritable bowel syndrome.[138]

Bennett[139] concluded that fibromyalgia and MPS may be two distinct entities which may have the same underlying pathophysiology, as there are many similarities between the two syndromes, including trigger points found in fibromyalgia patients. Similar to chronic tension-type headache, EMG findings in fibromyalgia are typically negative or equivocal concerning the correlation of muscle tension with pain.[139,140] No specific psychological findings are noted.[138,139] The sleep disturbance is similar to that seen in chronic tension-type headache and may be linked to a deficiency of serotonin.[141] Disturbances in oculomotor function are found in chronic tension-type headache, to a lessor degree than in fibromyalgia patients.[142,143] Sympathetic blockade has been found to diminish pain and decrease tender points, indicative of sympathetic hyperactivity and a related disturbance of microcirculation.[140,143,144] The sympathetic aspects seen in MPS and associated chronic tension-type headache have already been mentioned.[111,112] Similar to chronic tension-type headache, abnormalities of serotonin binding to platelets, a marker of central nervous system serotonergic efficacy, has also been found in fibromyalgia.[124,129]

Jay[145] analyzed three groups of 20 patients with chronic tension-type headache, with final diagnoses of chronic tension-type headache, myofascial pain syndrome, and fibromyalgia, on the basis of physical examination and published diagnostic criteria. A continuum of symptom severity in the three groups was seen, including progressively increasing affective and physical problems as age, time in pain, and severity increased. The findings were found to show a progression, less to more severe, from chronic tension-type headache to the MPS group and finally to the fibromyalgia group. The signs and symptoms of chronic tension-type headache were identified in the MPS and fibromyalgia groups. Localized trigger points were found in patients with simple tension-type headache.

Neurophysiological changes

Less than half of tension-type headache patients complain of mild associated autonomic symptoms such as lack of appetite, hyperirritability, dizziness, and increased light sensitivity.[146] Notably, some of these symptoms may be secondary to the autonomic changes associated with active myofascial trigger points located in the head and neck.

While muscle contraction and tenderness may be interpreted as primary symptoms of tension-type headache (TTHA), EMG activity and muscle tenderness increase more often during migraine than tension-type headache.[147–149]

In research comparing tension-type headache with common migraine patients exposed to auditory stimulation, TTHA patients showed a lower heart-rate reactivity than migraine patients.[150] Haynes[151] showed that TTHA patients exhibit the greatest cardiovascular arousal during headache. In another study,[99] both migraine and TTHA patients decreased pulse velocity in response to noise, while controls experienced increased pulse velocity. In a psychophysiological comparison of migraine and tension-type headache, Cohen[147] found that migraine patients are vasodilated and TTHA patients are vasoconstricted both during and between headache attacks. During another study, administration of ergotamine tartrate, a vasoconstrictor, increased the pain of tension-type headache, while amyl nitrate, a vasodilator, yielded only transient pain relief.[152]

A study by Murphy and Lehrer[114] indicated greater sympathetic arousal during tension-type headache as compared to controls. Another study[153] reported both TTHA and migraine patients demonstrated cardiovascular sympathetic hypofunction, indicated by low basal levels of norepinephrine as well as orthostatic hypotension. Covelli and Ferrannini[154] suggested that TTHA patients have phasic hypersympathetic activity, while migraineurs do not differ from controls during psychogalvanic response testing.

Evidence of pupillary sympathetic hypofunction and subtle anisocoria was found in both tension-type headache and migraine patients.[155] It was suggested that this may have reflected a central bioaminergic system dysfunction. Another study suggested a pupillary sympathetic system imbalance in chronic tension-type headache patients, who showed asymmetric mydriasis after tyramine instillation and in the physiologic pupillary tests.[156] Rosenhall et al.[142] noted oculomotor dysfunction in the amplitude and number of corrective saccades during testing of tension-type headache patients.

Drummond[157] noted increased photophobia in TTHA patients as compared to controls. He hypothesized that changes in central modulation may induce increased sensitivity or hyperexcitability-induced photophobia.

Episodic platelet abnormalities with associated serotonergic dysfunction has been well documented in migraine.[158,159] Decreased platelet serotonin in chronic tension-type headache patients has also been noted.[160]

Neuroanatomy and neurochemistry

Central modulation of pain appears to originate in the brainstem, involving at least two systems. The inhibitory "descending" analgesia system appears to regulate the spinal cord "gating" mechanisms. It includes the midbrain periaquaductal gray region, the medial medullary raphe nuclei and adjacent reticular formation, and the dorsal horn neurons of the spinal cord.[161] The "ascending" pain modulation system originates in the midbrain and projects to the thalamus.[162] Both systems heavily utilize biogenic amines, opioid peptides, and nonopioid peptides.[161–163]

The ascending system appears to be more relevant to headache disorders.[163] This system has a brainstem to (medial) thalamus projection which includes both serotonergic and opiate receptors in large numbers. The midbrain dorsal raphe nucleus, a serotonergic nucleus, projects to the medial thalamus and is associated with pain perception.[162] Raskin[164] has reviewed literature implicating serotonergic projections to the forebrain in sleep-cycle regulation, mood changes, pain perception, and the hypothalamic regulation of hormone release.

In the central nervous system (CNS), the endogenous opiate system (EOS) may act as a nociceptive "rheostat" or "algostat", setting pain modulation to a particular level. As this level changes, an individual's pain tolerance may also change. Fluctuations in the intensity of pain may be interpreted as being caused by fluctuations in the function of antinociceptive pathways.[165,166] Terenius[167] suggested that patients with chronic neuropathic pain, who have been noted to have low beta-endorphin levels, may be more prone to develop a pain syndrome caused not by excessive nociceptive stimulation, but rather by a deficiency in the EOS control mechanisms. Headache and other "non-organic" central pain problems are thought to be the most common expression of impairment of the antinociceptive systems.[168]

The endogenous opiates modulate the neurovegetative triad of pain, depression, and autonomic disturbances which are found in only two conditions: chronic tension-type headache and morphine abstinence.[168] They are also implicated as primary protagonists in idiopathic headache.[168,169] Reduced plasma concentrations of beta-endorphin have been found in idiopathic headache patients, including chronic tension-type headache.[170–173] Normal levels were found in one study.[174] Increased levels of beta-endorphin are found at the end of a headache attack, possibly associated with stress induced by the headache pain[175] and suggested by the fact that adrenocorticotropic hormone (ACTH) and beta-endorphin are located in the same hypothalamic neurons.

A primary relationship exists between the EOS and the biogenic amine systems. This relationship is intrinsic both to the pathophysiology of pain modulation and to the treatment. Clinical and pharmacological information indicates that dysmodulated serotonergic neurotransmission probably generates chronic headache and head pain. It has also been hypothesized that ordinary periodic headache may be the "noise" of serotonergic neurotransmission.[163]

Serotonergic uptake mechanisms in the platelet are similar to those of neurons.[176] Platelet serotonergic levels were found to be lower in patients with chronic tension-type headache as compared to controls.[160] Decreased levels of plasma serotonin were also found in chronic tension-type headache patients.[177] Shimomura and Takehashi[178] also found decreased levels of serotonin in the platelets of tension-type headache patients and, along with Giacovazzo et al.,[177] believe that this indicates a central serotonergic disturbance, possibly an impairment of serotonergic metabolism in patients with chronic tension-type headache.

Substance P, an excitatory neuropeptide, is found at all levels of the neuro-axis. Lower levels of substance P have been found in chronic neuropathic and idiopathic headache/pain patients than in normal volunteers.[179,180]

Platelet GABA levels in chronic tension-type headache patients are significantly increased compared to those seen in migraine patients and normal controls. Increased GABA levels may counterbalance neuronal hyperexcitability and may also be associated with depression.[181]

Low levels of plasma norepinephrine are found in both migraine and chronic tension-type headache patients in response to the cold pressor test, suggesting peripheral sympathetic hypofunction.[182] Noradrenergic dysfunction may also participate in the etiology or maintenance of central opioid dysfunction.[173]

Opioid receptor mechanisms are apparently very susceptible to desensitization, or the development of tolerance. In chronic tension-type headache sufferers, opioid receptor hypersensitivity is marked, probably because of the chronically diminished secretion of neurotransmitters. Sicuteri[183] called this the "empty neuron syndrome", indicating that it may involve both autonomic and nociceptive afferent systems, in addition to being latent, subpathological, or pathological with spontaneous manifestations.

The EOS modulates the activity of monoaminergic neurons. A chronic EOS deficiency can provoke transmitter leakage, both opioid and bioaminergic, leading to neuronal exhaustion and "emptying", as well as compensatory effector cell hypersensitivity. The most important phenomena of the hypoendorphin syndromes would appear to be the poor release of transmitter and cell/receptor hypersensitivity.[168] Langemark et al.[105] also concluded that chronic tension-type headache may result from a dysmodulation of nociceptive impulses, with sensitized receptors also being involved.

Chronic idiopathic headache, such as chronic tension-type headache, may therefore be a "pain disease" linked to central dysmodulation of the nociceptive and antinociceptive systems, either latent or pathological in nature. Research indicates that at least two arms of the main endogenous antinociceptive systems, the EOS and the serotonergic system, are involved in the pathogenesis of chronic tension-type headache. This problem appears to be progressive, but it is uncertain as to whether the dysfunctions result from a genetic deficiency or neuronal exhaustion secondary to continuous activation of the systems.[172,183]

Pathophysiology of chronic tension-type headache

Figure 9 summarizes the pathophysiological mechanisms of chronic tension-type headache. Continuous peripheral stimulation from myofascial nociceptive input may effectively trigger a change in the central pain "rheostat" associated with nociceptive input, secondary to the continuous need for

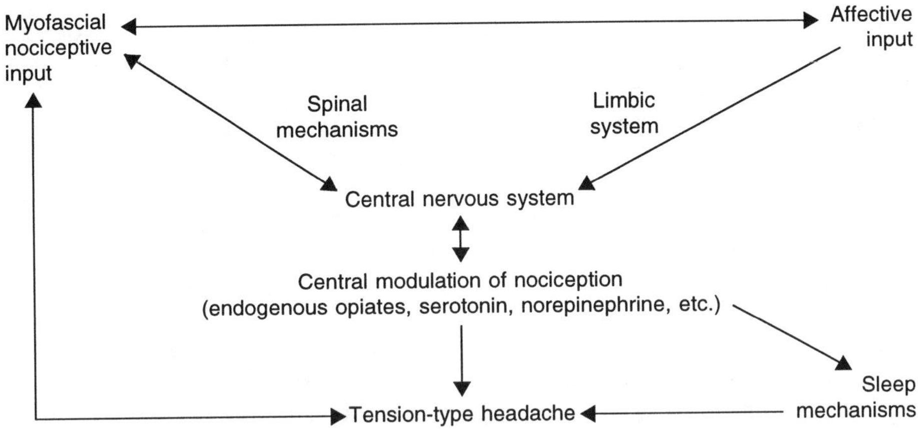

Figure 9 Pathophysiology of chronic daily or chronic tension-type headache. (From Jay, G.W., in *Treating the Headache Patient,* Cady, R.K. and Fox, A.W. (Eds.) Marcel Dekker, New York, 1995, pp. 211–233. With permission.)

pain-modulating, antinociceptive neurotransmitters. The affective aspects of pain, secondary to changes in neurotransmitters such as serotonin and which include depression, anxiety, and fear, can directly influence myofascial nociception, as well as further reinforce central neurochemical changes.

After 2 to 4 months (possibly sooner in some patients), changes in the central nervous system's central modulation of nociception can occur. Following continuous peripheral nociceptive stimulation, in association with affective changes, the central modulating mechanisms will assume a primary rather than a secondary or reactive role in pain perception, as well as antinociception, shifting pain perception initiation from the peripheral regions to the central nervous system.

This shift may make innocuous stimuli more aggravating to the pain-modulating systems. These already "dysmodulated" internal feedback mechanisms may react until central neurochemical mechanisms dominate, secondary to neurotransmitter exhaustion, and receptor hypersensitivity and abnormal biogenic amine metabolism/exhaustion occurs. As previously discussed, the intrinsic neurochemical changes may induce and/or exacerbate a sleep disorder, which by itself may perpetuate the central neurochemical dysmodulation which is primarily responsible for chronic tension-type headache.

Chronic post-traumatic tension-type headache, associated with a minor traumatic brain injury (MTBI) or not, has the same pathophysiological mechanisms. In the presence of a MTBI there is the addition of (1) direct myofascial trauma, (2) diffuse axonal injury, which also affects the neurochemistry of the brain as neuronal degeneration and death occurs, and (3) excitotoxic injury leading to cell death from over-exuberant production of acetylcholine and glutamate.[207] Affective changes typically follow, with the additional problem of possible cognitive changes resulting from a minor traumatic brain injury. The latter may make treatment more difficult, as treatment must involve patient education. Post-traumatic tension-type headache is the most common sequellae of a minor traumatic brain injury. It may be associated with iatrogenic analgesic abuse. Before treatment of cognitive deficit is attempted, inappropriate medications must be stopped and the headache ameliorated.

Migraine and tension-type headache: two entities?

Much has been written about transformational headache, where an episodic migraine may transform into chronic tension-type headache, or migraine may arise from episodic tension-type headache. There is no question that chronic tension-type headache may evolve from episodic tension-type headache, as the former is an extension and result of central changes induced over time by the latter.

It has been shown that chronic tension-type headache is associated with systemic changes in serotonin metabolism as well as changes in the EOS and various other neurotransmitters and peptides. Migraine itself has associated serotonergic changes, possibly associated with EOS changes, which are not long lasting and do not appear to be secondary to a dysmodulation of the basic nociceptive/antinociceptive neurochemical substrates.

Rather than migraine and acute and chronic tension-type headache being at the two extremes of a headache continuum, it appears that both entities are different manifestations of the neurochemical/neurophysiological dysmodulation of central pain modulating systems. Migraine is episodic in nature, with seemingly specific, self-limited neurophysiological and neurochemical changes. Chronic tension-type headache is associated with neurochemical changes which appear to be continuous, multifaceted, and similar in nature to those changes seen in other chronic pain syndromes, from pain arising from various places in the body. This appears to be true at least for those pain syndromes with myofascial/musculoskeletal etiologies, as differentiated from deafferentation-induced neurochemical and neurophysiological changes. Perhaps, when looked at from this perspective, diagnosis, as well as treatment, can be more easily identified and routinely implemented.

chapter six

Evaluation and treatment of tension-type headache

As previously noted, the neurological examination of migraine patients is, in the absence of complicated aura, negative. The examination of the cluster headache patient may yield signs of a partial Horner's syndrome. The examination of the patient with tension-type headache may yield a great deal of information.

Typically, the neurological examination is negative. It is the musculoskeletal evaluation that will give you the facts. Begin by observing the patient's shoulders. In the vast majority of cases, there is an asymmetry of the acromioclavicular joints, with one being higher than the other secondary to greater ipsilateral muscle spasm. The large muscles should be carefully palpated both for general tenderness and the presence of trigger points. These include the trapezius muscles, the deltoids, the scalenes, the rhomboids, the levaeter scapulae, and all associated muscles, including the pericranial musculature. Pay careful attention to the sternocleidomastoid muscles, particularly in patients complaining of dizziness and tinnitus. Palpate the bioccipital and bitemporal insertions. Look for true pericranial muscle tenderness, as well as masseter pain or tenderness. Observe the patient opening his mouth; look for the amount of space between the teeth and see if the jaw deviates.

Perform the passive as well as active cervical range of motion. Observe the patient's head — is it flexed forward? Is it tilted to one side? What about the shoulders — are they rounded? Rolled forward? Evaluate the presence and degree of muscle spasm found in the paravertebral muscles over the entire length of the spine.

If the patient is a chronic tension-type headache sufferer or if there is a complaint of upper extremity or hand numbness, perform an axillary stretch maneuver as well as the Adson's maneuver to evaluate for a myogenic thoracic outlet syndrome. And those are just the basics.

Until you know what you are dealing with physiologically, it is impossible to determine an appropriate treatment plan. Once you know and are positive about your diagnosis (reached by the history and physical/neurological examination), you can begin to formulate a treatment plan.

Treatment of episodic tension-type headache

The medical management of acute, episodic tension-type headache is relatively easy. Remember that the older nomenclature titled these headaches as "acute muscle contraction headache" or "tension headache". This form of headache is the most common, as previously indicated, accounting for up to 80% of all nonorganic types of headache. It has been estimated that over 90% of Americans experience an acute tension-type headache at some time. The majority of these headaches are self treated with over-the-counter medications and therefore never come to the attention of a physician. This indicates that the statistics are probably low, in that a fairly large number go unnoticed by physicians.

The greatest problem in the treatment of acute tension-type headache is the avoidance of the development of analgesic rebound headache, which can easily occur if a patient is over-medicated. This is one step into the development of chronic or daily tension-type headache. Physicians should be particularly familiar with the various types of medications which can be utilized for patients complaining of occasional tension-type headache.

The old adage, that less is better, certainly applies here. Many patients deal with the pain and discomfort by taking two aspirin and relaxing. Exercise is useful, as is a simple glass of wine, on an occasional basis. Any type of relaxation which distracts the patient from his headache is useful.

Dealing with the medication management, physicians have a more than ample supply of medications from which to choose. It may therefore be tempting to over-treat a minor headache with medications that have a significant risk of dependency. So be careful out there!

The simple analgesics are easily chosen by the patient, if not the physician. They are inexpensive and easy to get. They include aspirin and acetaminophen. Like the nonsteroidal antiinflammatory drugs (NSAIDs), aspirin appears to work by inhibiting the synthesis of prostaglandin by blocking the action of cyclooxygenase, an enzyme which enables the conversion of arachidonic acid to prostaglandin. Remember that prostoglandins are synthesized from cellular membrane phospholipids after activation or injury, and they sensitize pain receptors.

Aspirin, the prototypical NSAID, has antiinflammatory and antipyretic properties along with its pain-relieving properties. The recommended adult dose for treatment of acute tension-type headache is 650 mg every 6 hours. Gastric irritation may be decreased by taking the aspirin with milk or food. Aspirin can also double bleeding time for 4 to 7 days after taking as little as

.65 grams. Peak blood levels are found after 45 minutes. The plasma half-life is 2 to 30 hours.

Acetaminophen usage is common. It provides about the same amount of analgesia as aspirin but does not have the gastrointestinal side effects. That acetaminophen may work by inhibition of prostaglandin synthesis in the central nervous system has been suggested. It has much weaker antiinflammatory activity than aspirin. Peak plasma levels occur between 30 and 60 minutes. Its plasma half-life is 2 to 4 hours.

Ibuprofen, an NSAID, is also available over the counter in doses of 200 mg per tablet. It can cause significant gastrointestinal distress. It has a half-life of 2 to 4 hours, with peak plasma levels attained in 1 to 2 hours. The adult dosage is 200 to 400 mg every 4 to 6 hours, with a maximum of 1200 mg per day.

These medications are frequently sold in combination with other drugs such as caffeine, which exerts no specific analgesic effects but may potentiate the analgesic effects of aspirin and acetaminophen. There are aspirin-caffeine combination drugs (Anacin) and aspirin, acetaminophen, and caffeine combinations (Excedrin Extra-Strength and Vanquish). The recommended dosage is two tablets every 6 hours as needed.

The biggest problem is that taking aspirin, acetaminophen, or combination tablets daily or even every other day for a week or more (possibly less) can induce the problem of analgesic rebound headache (which will be discussed later).

As with birth control pills, when you ask a patient what medications they are taking, they may forget that the birth control pill or aspirin or acetaminophen are medications. Thus, they will forget to tell you about them, or they may even be too embarrassed to tell you because they are taking a large number of pills each day. So, be certain to ask specifically.

A number of NSAIDs are prescribed. Because of the variability in their efficacy, pharmacokinetics, and side effects, patients may need to be tried on more than one (sequentially, not in combination) to determine the best one for them.

The NSAIDs work, as noted before, by interfering with the action of cyclooxygenase in the synthesis of prostoglandins. Gastrointestinal side effects are common and occur in up to 15 to 20% of patients. These side effects may include epigastric pain, nausea, heartburn, and abdominal discomfort. A history of gastrointestinal bleeding or ulcerations should indicate that great caution must be used, if these medications are used at all.

The most frequently prescribed NSAIDs include:

- Naproxen sodium (Anaprox), which reaches peak plasma levels in 1 to 2 hours and has a mean half-life of 13 hours. It can be taken at 275 or 550 mg every 6 to 8 hours, with a top dosage of 1375 mg per day. Remember that this NSAID is useful in treating hormonally related migraine.

- Ibuprofen (Motrin), which is prescribed in dosages of 600 and 800 mg per tablet. The suggested dosage for mild to moderate pain is 400 mg every 4 to 6 hours as needed.
- Ketoprofen (Orudis), which is this author's NSAID of choice. It is a cyclooxygenase inhibitor but also stabilizes lysosomal membranes and possibly antagonizes the actions of bradykinin. Its peak plasma level is reached in 1 to 2 hours, and it has a 2-hour plasma half-life. It is now available over the counter (12.5-mg tablets) but is best used as 50- to 75-mg capsules. The recommended daily dosage is 150 to 300 mg a day in three or four divided doses. Gastrointestinal side effects are generally mild. Care should be taken when it is being given to a patient with impaired renal function.
- Ketorolac tromethamine (Toradol), which is a relatively new NSAID. It can be given orally or parenterally for moderate to severe acute headache pain. Peak plasma levels occur after intramuscular injection in about 50 minutes. Its analgesic effect is considered to be roughly equivalent to a 10-mg dose of intramuscular morphine. The typical injectable dose is 60 mg. Because of its potentially significant hepatic/renal side effects, the FDA has stated that Toradol should be given orally, after an intramuscular injection of 60 mg, at a dose of 10 mg every 8 hours for a maximum of 5 days.

Muscle relaxants are given for acute tension-type headache by some clinicians. They are probably best utilized during the first 3 weeks after onset of injury-related headache. They are useful in patients with significant muscle spasm and pain, which is not usually seen with episodic tension-type headache. They are used appropriately upon development of muscle spasm after injury such as a slip and fall, motor vehicle accident, work or athletic injuries, or overstretching.

These medications work via the development of a therapeutic plasma level. Their exact mechanism of action is unknown, but they do not directly affect striated muscle, the myoneural junction, or motor nerves. They produce relaxation by depressing the central nerve pathways, possibly through their effects on higher CNS centers, which modify the central perception of pain without affecting the peripheral pain reflexes or motor activity.

Carisoprodol (Soma) is a CNS depressant which metabolizes into a barbiturate, which makes it both addictive and particularly inappropriate to use for patients with pain from muscle spasm and minor traumatic brain injury. It acts as a sedative and is thought to depress polysynaptic transmission in interneuronal pools at the supraspinal level in the brainstem reticular formation. It is short lived, with peak plasma levels in 1 to 2 hours and a half-life of 4 to 6 hours. Dosage is 350 mg every 6 to 8 hours. It should not be mixed with other CNS depressants. For additional analgesic effects, it is also marketed in two other combined forms: with aspirin (as Soma Compound) and with codeine.

Chlorzoxazone (Parafon Forte DSC) is a centrally acting muscle relaxant with fewer sedative properties. It inhibits the reflex arcs involved in producing and maintaining muscle spasm at the level of the spinal cord and subcortical areas of the brain. It reaches it peak plasma level in 3 to 4 hours, and duration of action is 3 to 4 hours. It is well tolerated, and side effects are uncommon. Dosage is 500 mg three times a day.

Metaxalone (Skelaxin) is a centrally acting skeletal muscle relaxant which is chemically related to mephenaxalone, a mild tranquilizer. It is thought to induce muscle relaxation via CNS depression. Onset of action is about 1 hour, with peak blood levels in 2 hours. Duration of action is 4 to 6 hours. The recommended dose is 2400 to 3200 mg a day in divided doses (tablets are 400 mg each). It should be used carefully in patients with impaired liver function and should not be used at all in patients with significant renal or liver disease in addition to a history of drug-induced anemias. Side effects include nausea, vomiting, gastrointestinal upset, drowsiness, dizziness, headache, nervousness, and irritability, as well as rash or pruritis. Jaundice and hemolytic anemia are rare.

Methocarbamol (Robaxin, Robaxisal) is a centrally acting skeletal muscle relaxant. It may inhibit nerve transmission in the internuncial neurons of the spinal cord. It has a 30-minute onset of action. Peak levels are found in about 2 hours, and its duration of action is 4 to 6 hours. It comes as 500-and 750-mg tablets. Tablets containing methocarbamol and aspirin (Robaxisal) are also available. The recommended dose of Robaxin is 750 mg three times a day. As with all of these medications, it should be taken for 7 to 10 days. It is well tolerated, with initial side effects which resolve over time and which include lightheadedness, dizziness, vertigo, headache, rash, gastrointestinal upset, nasal congestion, fever, blurred vision, urticaria, and mild muscular incoordination. In situations of severe, seemingly intractable muscle spasm, Robaxin may be given intravenously in doses of about a gram every 8 to 12 hours.

Orphenedrine citrate (Norflex, Norgesic) is a centrally acting skeletal muscle relaxant with anticholinergic properties thought to work by blocking neuronal circuits, the hyperactivity of which may be implicated in hypertonia and spasm. It is available in injectable and oral formulations. The intramuscular dose of Norflex is 2 mg, while the intravenous dosage is 60 mg in aqueous solution. The oral formulation (Norflex) is given in 100-mg tablets, one tablet every 12 hours. Norgesic is a combination form that includes caffeine and aspirin, and 1 or 2 tablets should be given every 6 to 8 hours. Norgesic Forte, a stronger combination, is given in doses of one half to one tablet every 6 to 8 hours. Because of its anticholinergic effects, it should be contraindicated in patients with glaucoma, prostatic enlargement, or bladder outlet obstruction. Its major side effects are also secondary to its anticholinergic properties and include tachycardia, palpitations, urinary retention, nausea, vomiting, dizziness, constipation, and drowsiness. It may also cause confusion, excitation, hallucinations, and syncope.

Many of these medications are given in combination with other drugs, including barbiturates (butalbatal and meprobamate) and narcotics (codeine, oxycodone, propoxyphene, etc.) This is probably not a good idea, as the barbiturates and narcotics can easily lead to patient dependence.

A good combination utilized by the author is methocarbamol, 750 mg three times a day for 10 days in patients with significant spasm, accompanied by ketoprofen, 75 mg every 6 to 8 hours as needed, with food as needed. For the occasional (episodic) tension-type headache, one tablet of each taken together every 6 to 8 hours for two to three doses works very well. Again, narcotic medications should not be used for the patient with acute or episodic tension-type headache, as the risk of dependence is too great.

Remember, too, that simple acute tension-type headache is a problem that the headache specialists are rarely called in to see. It is the patient's family physician or chiropractor who most frequently sees this problem.

Medication management of chronic tension-type headache

In this section we are looking at the medication management of patients with chronic tension-type headache without a true vascular headache component. We will look at the treatment of combination headache later. The medication treatment of choice is the tricyclic antidepressants (TCAs) or the specific serotonin re-uptake inhibitors (SSRIs).

The particular TCA medication of choice is amitriptyline, a sedating tricyclic antidepressant. Like all of the tricyclics, it works in the synapse to decrease re-uptake of serotonin and (depending on the individual medication) norepinephrine. Amitriptyline, unlike the other TCAs, also works to repair the damage in stage 4 sleep architecture. It is the most sedating tricyclic. The typical dosage is between 10 and 50 mg at night. The author has found it rare to need more than 20 or 30 mg at night.

> **AH HA!** *Now to say something bad — that is, something that will typically get you in trouble with a managed care company which gives you their medication formulary. When using psychoactive medications it has been my long experience that generics do not work as well as the "real stuff".*

Do I say that just to be difficult? Not at all! In several unpublished studies, performed at multiple headache centers, it was noted that Elavil was better than amitriptyline. How did we know this? Magic? No, we gave all patients a headache calendar, along with their Elavil. When they returned for re-evaluation, their calendars were pretty blank. When a patient came back with a marked increase in headache, it was found in over 90% of the patients that they had been given amitriptyline by their pharmacist, not Elavil. To clinch the topic, when they were started again on Elavil, within a month, the number of their headaches fell again to almost nothing.

The idea that generics are the total equivalent to non-generics is, unfortunately, just not true, particularly when dealing with psychotropics as well as anticonvulsants. Remember the old Parke-Davis Dilantin Cap Seals? Well, patients would take three at bedtime (300 mg) and because of the pharmacokinetics and bioavailability profile, they would remain seizure free. Then came the world of generics. Patients who took their dilantin at night began to have seizure during the day. Why? The generics had phenytoin, but also had different pharmacokinetics and bioavailability.

To make matters worse, when a pharmacy runs out of its generic medication amitriptyline, it sends out a bid to different suppliers who will sell them amitriptyline. The bid goes, typically, to the lowest bidder, *but* each generic supplier's amitriptyline has at least slightly different pharmacokinetics and bioavailability, meaning it will work a bit differently each time, even though it is the "same" drug. How tightly it is packed, the other components of the tablet, etc. all make a difference. So, even if you cannot get the non-generic, it is problematic that the patient will get the same generic each time, or even most of the time.

Neuropharmacologically, this is not good — not that anyone really cares except us folk in the trenches and the patients who may get suboptimal treatment. To make matters still worse, managed care companies, HMOs, and their new formularies can now make substitutions whenever or however they want. If you order ketoprofen for your patient, for example, your patient's managed care company or HMO is able to substitute ibuprofen for your prescription, even if you know that your patient has tried it and it did not help. You then have to call or write the formulary committee or the medical director to try to get your patient the medication that you, their physician, wants him to have.

Now, if only physicians would band together and do something about stuff like this, we would really be helping our patients, as well as ourselves. Do you want to be sued for a severe side effect of a drug automatically substituted for the medication you prescribed? Ahhh, the Impossible Dream.

Getting back to the subject at hand, doxepin is a very good tricyclic. Anticholinergic side effects such as sedation are reduced (but not by much) when compared to amitriptyline. It does not work on the sleep architecture. It is used at the same dosage levels of amitriptyline.

Notice that the tricyclics are not used in their antidepressant dosages, which can vary from 100 to 350 mg a day. Even though the doses are low, their effectiveness in the treatment of chronic tension-type headache is apparent.

The SSRIs include Prozac, Paxil, and Zoloft. These medication are not typically sedating, although for some patients they may be, and with the exclusion of such patients they are energizing. They should be given in the morning. Prozac and Paxil should start at 10 to 20 mg a day, and they can be increased to 60 to 80 mg. Zoloft should be given at 25 to 50 mg in the morning, up to 150 mg in divided doses. You should divide the doses, giving one when the patient gets up in the morning (around 7:00 a.m.) and one at noon. Explain to the patients that taking these medications later than noon can, in many cases, give them problems sleeping. You can also safely combine 10 to 40 mg of Prozac or Paxil or 50 mg of Zoloft with a small dose of amitriptyline or doxepin (10 to 30 mg) at night. There are other excellent antidepressants, such as Wellbuterin, Serzone, and Effexor. These should be considered as needed. Do not combine these medications with the monoamine oxidase (MAO) inhibitors. It is just not a great idea.

Another excellent medication is clonazepam, a fifth-generation form of benzodiazepine. It is GABAnergic in effect. It works at the level of the internuncial neurons of the spinal cord to enhance muscle relaxation. It helps, a bit, with anxiolysis. It has a side effect of sedation. In doses of 4 to 12 mg a day, it works as an anticonvulsant. At smaller doses, .5 to 1 mg given at night, it is very useful in the treatment of patients with chronic tension-type headache. The sedation lasts for a shorter time than the sedation from tricyclics, and this in itself is useful.

> **AH HA!** *Here's the easiest way to save your patients grief and their insurance companies money which would be (and should not be) spent unnecessarily. Are you ready? Treating patients with chronic tension-type headache with tricyclics, physical therapy, psychotherapy, etc.,* ***will not work if the patient is taking daily or four times a week analgesic medications of any type!*** *Ta-daahhh! It's a big, major, money-saving secret, which the vast majority of clinicians do not know, or ignore if they do know. So, you can be a hero to the patient's managed care company or HMO by taking him off of analgesics before you do any other treatment. Now you know!*

Cost-effective treatment of chronic tension-type headache

Treatment of chronic tension-type headache is best accomplished via an interdisciplinary rehabilitation approach, the main purpose of which is *not* to teach the patient to live with the headache, but rather to diagnose the patient's headache properly and ameliorate or stop it. Drug detoxification is the necessary first step, whether the patient is over-utilizing simple, over-the-counter analgesics or narcotics or barbiturates. Chronic daily analgesics appear to prevent appropriate functioning of the EOS (via negative neurochemical feedback loops) and other associated antinociceptive systems, inducing analgesic rebound headaches which are secondary problems from the medications which induce headache secondary to purely neurochemical/neurophysiological changes. Vascular rebound headaches from over-utilization of vasoconstrictors may also occur and must be stopped before other treatment is applied. Clinically, an effective way to detoxify chronic tension-type headache patients is with the repetitive DHE-45 protocol described by Raskin.[164] Concurrently, prophylactic medications should be started. The use of prophylactic medications, as well as physical therapy and other treatments given while a patient is enduring analgesic rebound headaches, is an ineffectual waste of time and money.

After detoxification, an outpatient interdisciplinary headache rehabilitation program utilizing neuropharmacological therapy (to restore neurochemical homeostasis), physical therapy,[184] psychotherapy, and stress management (including biofeedback-enhanced neuromuscular re-education and muscle relaxation) is the most time- and cost-effective treatment. Optimal psychotherapy or physical therapy regimes by themselves will not resolve myofascial difficulties or depression if the affective, sleep, and central nervous system neurochemical dysmodulation affecting them is not concurrently and appropriately treated. The interdisciplinary treatment paradigm also enables fine-tuning of diagnosis and possible determination of a secondary or "hidden" etiology for a patient's headaches.

Failure to treat the chronic tension-type headache patient with an interdisciplinary, whole-person approach (see Figure 9 in Chapter 5) is responsible for multiple treatment failures as well as monetary waste, as long-term response — headache remediation — is most often not achieved.

Next, we will talk about the diagnosis and treatment of combination headache and I will give you some more AH HA!s. You, too, can become a headache maven, and you are more than half of the way there!

chapter seven

Combination headache

The most common patient seen in clinical practice is the one with more than one type of headache. These patients have frequently seen many other clinicians and still complain of headaches, most typically daily. These patients may be difficult to manage, as they may present as angry, having seen so many other doctors who state that they will "fix" the problem. They are angry because the problem is still there, and they are still suffering. To make matters worse, although the patients may not know it, they are probably victims of iatrogenic medication addiction, even if they are not taking mostly narcotics.

Case study

A 38-year-old, righthanded male was seen in consultation. He developed headache 3 years earlier after being struck in the right forehead with a piece of metal. He had been seen by a "headache specialist" who had no specialized training. This "expert" started him on self-injected DHE-45 daily. He was then placed on not one, not two, but three antihypertensives to bring down his "high blood pressure" which was really there as a secondary effect of the typical autonomic responses to pain. He was then placed on narcotics for his pain, and finally two other vasoconstrictors. He was self-injecting DHE-45 2 days a week and sumatriptan 2 days a week and was taking Midrin 2 days a week. About 6 months before I saw him, he had an episode of orthostatic hypotension secondary to three antihypertensives and three vasoconstrictors. He fell flat on his face, which caused cervical trauma, which induced two ruptured cervical discs. He underwent surgery — cervical laminectomies at two levels and a fusion. When I saw him, he was, for obvious reasons, angry. He did not understand why he was still having so much pain.

> The first things — history, examination, and diagnosis — revealed a number of problems: right supraorbital neuropathy, cervical myofascial pain syndrome, analgesic rebound headache, vascular rebound headache, unilateral myogenic thoracic outlet syndrome, depression, anxiety disorder, and hypertension. **It should also be noted that taking an ergot within 24 hours of sumatriptan may cause cardiac problems.** But, what the hey, no one had ever mentioned this to the patient, who was self-injecting like mad to try to stop his headache pain.
>
> The first thing that was done was to get rid of all the vasoconstrictors, which in and of themselves can produce hypertension. Next, we got rid of the analgesics. Then, we cut down his antihypertensives to one, verapamil. We then treated the cervical myofascial pain syndrome and the myogenic thoracic outlet syndrome with physical therapy and his depression and anxiety with psychotherapy and biofeedback therapy. He was placed on a serotonergic antidepressant.
>
> Then, we found that his blood pressure was normal, so we stopped the verapamil. He had no headache, but he did have continued pain from the supraorbital neuralgia, which we dealt with by using a cryolytic procedure. He then had no pain, hypertension, depression, anxiety, myofascial pain syndrome, or neuralgic pain, which appeared to be his initial problem.
>
> Misdiagnosis and poor treatment by the original, self-proclaimed "headache specialist" created the majority of his initial diagnoses, the hypotensive episode, and the surgery required after it, as well as producing analgesic and vascular rebound headache and placing him in jeopardy by inappropriate medication usage.

The bottom line is that if you do not know what to do, do nothing yourself and send your patient for help or seek a second opinion by a true headache specialist. Yes, this patient was a tough one, but correct diagnosis at the onset and conservative medication management were the missing keys that would have helped the patient. The combination headache I found was secondary to iatrogenic medication abuse. Yes, the physician did it. And many clinicians do it, totally unknowingly, just trying to do their best to help their patients.

For the patient with combination headache, diagnosis is everything. You have to understand all the stuff in the first six chapters to do it correctly. Even then, there is more you need to know to do it right. First, how do you diagnose a patient with combination headache? Carefully, and, if you have the correct knowledge base, relatively easily. You take a history which, in over 95% of cases, will give you the diagnosis. Then you examine the patient carefully. You must rule out other neurological or organic causes of headache (see later in this book) before you are left with a primary headache diagnosis. By evaluating the patient's medication (that history thing) you can easily see if analgesic or vascular rebound is occurring. That being done correctly, you can make your initial diagnosis.

Will all of a patient's diagnoses be immediately obvious to you? Possibly not. If a patient is complaining of severe headaches every day, and you can find the myofascial reasons for daily headache, as well as the drug-related reasons, does that rule out migraine? Nope. It doesn't. Patients with combination headache are like onions, with multiple layers of problems. You might get through a number of layers of diagnosis at the onset, but that may not get you through all of the layers of problems.

When you treat a patient with a long, complex history that has been muddied by treatment by multiple clinicians and the patient is still having headache, what do you do? Start at the beginning. Take the patient off of all non-essential medications, in a physiological manner. That will deal with the analgesic and vascular rebound headaches. Try to undo whatever you can. Then start again, taking another history and doing another examination, if need be.

If you get a patient without all of the past baggage, but your treatment protocols do not work after 4 or 5 weeks and you do not know why, start again with another history and examination. There might be something you missed. Do not just throw more medications or therapies at patients in a shotgun approach.

You need to treat with a 38-caliber pharmacologic bullet, not a widespread pattern of shotgun pellets. Use one bullet for each diagnosis. The smartest way to do this is to treat what is obvious to you. If a patient has chronic tension-type headaches and analgesic and/or vascular rebound headache, treat those things first. Then see what, if anything, is left. After the daily headaches and the drug-related headaches are vanquished, you may find true migraine. Then, you treat the migraine by abortive or prophylactic methods, depending on the number of migraine headaches the patient experiences over a month or two. Yes, it may take two or more steps, and it may take a month or three, but you do it right the first time. The patient will thank you for it, too.

Your history should include the type of pain, the frequency of pain, and the severity of pain, as well as its typical duration. The type of pain is important. Does it feel like burning? Or does it feel like lancinating (like an electrical shock)? Is there a single place where it is constantly present? Is there another place or places where you can touch and cause the shooting, burning, electrical-like pain to occur? A "yes" answer to any of these questions means you should be looking for a neuropathic pain problem, such as trigeminal neuralgia or a peripheral nerve neuropathy ... or even a cranial nerve neuropathy (more on these later on, don't get anxious!).

The pain of migraine is considered to be throbbing and to be unilateral in the majority of adults. But not all. There can be bilateral migraine. Ask if the patient had a history of childhood migraine. Car sickness? Cyclic vomiting or abdominal pain? If the answer is "yes", consider this. Pediatric migraine is bilateral in the majority of cases. One third of the patients lose their headaches when they reach puberty. One third become the typical unilateral migraine headache sufferers. And one third continue to have bilateral migraine.

Another problem with the myth of unilateral headache being migraine is that an acute, unilateral muscle spasm or cervical strain/sprain may bring on an acute, one-sided headache with throbbing pain. It may be associated with photophobia and even nausea, possibly vomiting. (These are pretty general autonomic signs of head pain.) Yet, it is not a migraine, and treating it with a vasoconstrictor will not help. Treating it with an NSAID, such as intramuscular Toradol, may.

The point is, it may look and smell like a migraine and not be one. It may look like anything and not be what you think it is. You have to take the history and examine the patient yourself.

The pain of tension-type headache is described as a tight, aching pain, vice-like, like a tight bathing cap, etc. So, you see a patient who tells you they had a visual aura, followed by severe, throbbing, unilateral pain associated with photo- and phonophobia, as well as nausea and vomiting. The patient was in so much pain that it was impossible to come in to see you yesterday, when this happened. Today the patient has less throbbing but more of a vice-like pain which starts at the sub-occipital regions. What is the diagnosis?

Well, we know that migraine with aura is what the patient described. So be it. But why the tension-type aspects? When we have a headache, we tend to protect ourselves from further head pain by splinting our head with our neck muscles, just like you would splint your arm with your other arm if you hurt it. So, after a true migraine, with or without aura, it is common to see the residual pain from a secondary tension-type headache — secondary to the patient's splinting their head by contracting their cervical muscles to prevent it from "flopping around" and causing more pain. When the migraine is over, the muscle spasm which reflexively occurred can still cause headache pain, but a different type of headache pain that is not migrainous headache pain. Treat it with an NSAID, if the patient can tolerate an NSAID, and move on. The sound of hoof beats outside the window more often comes from horses, not zebras. Just know your pathophysiology.

The pain description of cluster headache, as well as chronic paroxysmal hemicrania (CPH), does not sound like anything else, although you have to rule out neuropathy before you come to the diagnosis of CPH. Or, you can treat the patient with indomethacin. If the patient has total relief within 12 to 24 hours, you have made your diagnosis of CPH.

While it may sound like there are a lot of "pure" headache cases and associated causes running in and out of your office, there are not. You have to dig into each case individually, beginning with the history and examination. You can (and will) at least initially be fooled. What sounds straightforward may not be.

A patient tells you about their headache. You examine them and diagnose chronic tension-type headache. You treat them with a serotonergic medication. You give them physical therapy. Three weeks go by, and the patient is still complaining about daily headaches. Did you mess up? Misdiagnose the headache? Mistreat it? Maybe. Maybe not.

The body, particularly the brain, is like an engine — like the engine in your car, but about a million times more complicated. Yet, certain things in this analogy hold true. If you disconnect the distributor cap, the car won't run. If you put the wires back correctly, it will. The brain can be looked at like that, in a limited fashion. If a patient has myogenic nociception which induces headache, and if you rid the patient of that problem, as well as any associated affective problems he might have (depression, anxiety, etc.), then he should be better, right? Of course!

But what else can cause the daily headaches to continue if you have nailed the correct diagnosis and treated it appropriately? Obviously something else. During the history, you, of course, asked the patient about concurrent analgesic drug use. The patient said he was not taking anything else. From experience, let it be known that our patients are why we are in the healing business. But, sometimes, they do not tell you the whole, entire truth.

If you have a good relationship with your patient, the one described immediately above, you need to sit him down and ask again about medications, specifically including aspirin and acetaminophen. If the patient is antagonistic, get a urine for an analgesic panel, qualitative and quantitative. Sometimes patients do not realize that the over-the-counter analgesics are "really medications". Sometimes they are afraid to stop them, for fear that they will lose the "one thing that helps their headaches". Other times, they may be getting analgesics from another physician. On and on, *ad nauseum*.

So, back to the car analogy, if you connect all the wires back the correct way, the engine will run. If you treat the patient correctly for the proper diagnosis, the patient will stop having daily headaches. If he does not, then something else is going on. Either you missed something significant or the patient is doing something you are not aware of, such as taking analgesics or vasoconstrictors. Otherwise, the engine would work correctly, as would the brain, at least in terms of treating the headaches.

Go back and take another history, asking more specifically about medications, even the simple analgesics. Get a urine for a coma panel. Call the patient's pharmacist and ask if any other clinician is prescribing analgesics. Sound like detective work? Well, it is. Remember that Sherlock Holmes was patterned after a prominent neurologist, Dr. Bell, who was personally known by Sir Arthur Conan Doyle.

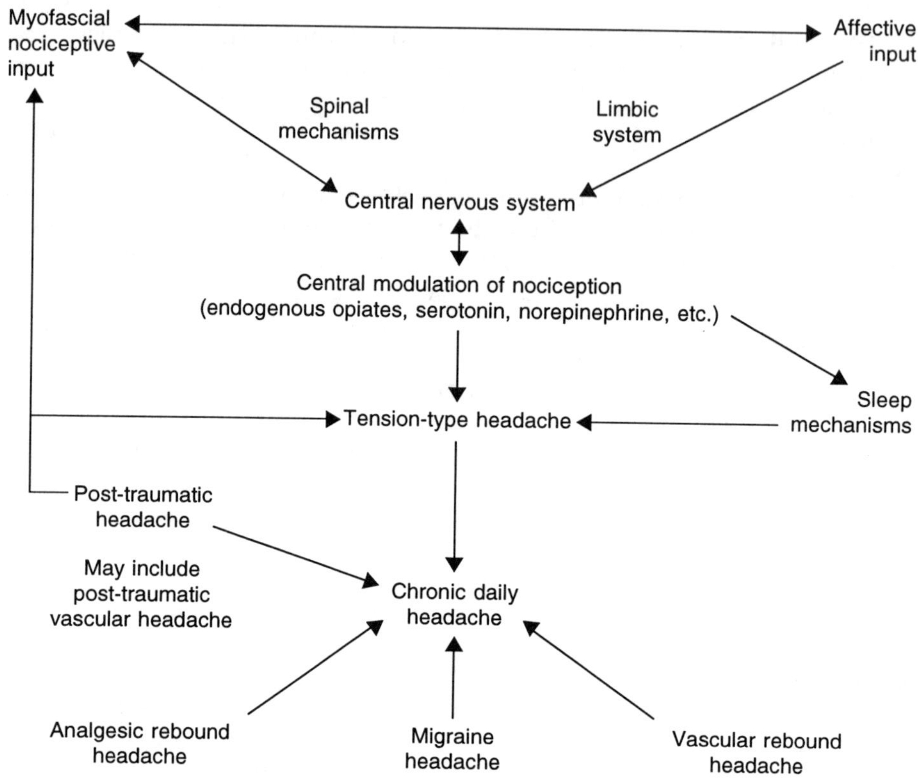

Figure 1 Pathophysiology of tension-type headache and chronic daily headache. (From Jay, G.W., *Pain Dig.*, 4:257, 1994. With permission.)

Remember also that most patients in the described situation are not trying to put something over on you. They truly may not understand what is going on, or why they should not take aspirin or something like it. But you know that if you do what is medically correct for the correct diagnosis, the result you should see is one in which the headache is ameliorated. If you do not see it happen, then something else is going on, and you have to find out what it is. That's your job. Just keep peeling back those onion layers. This is easy if you and your patient enjoy a good therapeutic relationship. Try your best to keep things calm and empathetic. You have to understand your patient, physically as well as emotionally and psychologically.

Figure 1 shows the relationship between tension-type headaches and chronic daily headaches. It should give you a good idea of the various types of headaches you should include or, more importantly, exclude from your headache diagnosis after all other organic/neurological problems have been ruled out.

In patients with a post-traumatic headache, be aware enough to at least consider the possibility of a mild traumatic brain injury or post-concussion syndrome (*not* the same things!). In the chapter on post-traumatic headaches, we will talk about the surprises that this additional diagnosis may give you, your patients, and their diagnosis of headache. The next chapter will discuss the psychology of headache. Or the psychology of the headache patient. Or, whatever. Just turn the page.

chapter eight

Psychological aspects of headache

One of the most frightening things that can occur to a patient with chronic headache is to be thought of as "crazy". Just asking patients to consider talking to a psychologist is tantamount to calling them crazy, from their perspective. Is that true? Are they crazy? Of course not.

But to many people, it is all right if you deal with an organic, physical illness; however, if you deal with their emotional status, that is definitely not all right. In Beverly Hills, CA, many well-to-do people may consider their psychological/psychoanalytic treatment as a measure of status. The majority of people, though, do not look at it like that. It is an intrusion into one's very being. It is not as though the headache is "just" in the patient's head, and if you, doctor, think it is, well, I will just go somewhere else to a better doctor. Remember several chapters back when we talked about serotonin. Decreases in serotonin due to chronic myofascial nociception may create depression. It is a chemical disorder. It is organic. It is real. If the patient has a sleep disorder, a change in appetite, and loss of libido, then he has the three neurovegetative signs of depression, which go along with the chemical changes in their brain.

Many people think of a depressed person as someone who sits in the corner crying. You need to explain that that perception is not correct. Depression is an organic problem, one that can hurt if it is not dealt with along with the other physical problems you have diagnosed.

A case study having nothing to do with headache

When I first entered practice, I was asked to see a very nice elderly woman with a history of chest pain going on for 4 years. It occurred twice a year at almost the same times. Each time it happened, she was hospitalized in the CCU (coronary care unit) and had a full cardiac work-up, as the pain was substernal and in

> every way mimicked a heart attack. Each time she had been hospitalized, her work-up was negative. Finally, pretty much out of desperation, her physician called in a pain specialist.
>
> Anyone who thinks I found a subtle cardiac problem missed by others is dead wrong. As a neurologist and pain medicine specialist, I do not do hearts. But, what I did was to take it from the top and take a general pain history. It was pretty much word for word what she had told her internist. There was nowhere for me to turn there, so, out of my own desperation, I asked her why she had pain twice a year and at the same time each year. This nice older woman looked at me like I was nuts and said, "That's when my husband died and when we unveiled his tombstone." Suddenly light dawned in the periphery of my vision.
>
> My next question was, of course, "How did your husband die?" Her answer, of course, was, "He had a heart attack." I immediately spoke with her internist, who was unaware of the correlation with her husband's death and why. Then I went through the patient's old charts. No one had ever asked her what she thought of her pain, or even why she had pain. The old anniversary reaction. Oy Vey!

This lovely woman taught me something important. Two things, actually. First, pain may have meaning, specific meaning. Second, to find out what it may be you have to ask. Ask specifically, even if you feel like a dummy.

An important differentiation to make is that between pain and suffering. If you have a tonically spasmed muscle with active trigger points or a needle lodged in your arm you will feel pain. When the muscle spasm is relieved or the pin has been removed, and full physiological healing occurs along with the return of a full range of motion, but the pain continues and you do not know why, on a physiological basis, that is typically considered suffering. Suffering is pain without organicity or abnormalities in the neurochemical milieu. It is the emotional and behavioral aspects of pain that have been learned over time, reinforced each day that the organic etiology of pain persisted. The typical patient will, of course, deny this. And why not? It is not a conscious process. It is learned.

Ever wonder why some women may have more severe pain during menses and complain about it (or not)? Research has shown that, too, is a learned behavior from when they were young and watched their mothers and older/younger sisters. If not family, who should you learn such things from — especially when it was perceived that your pain got you special consideration, such as not having to do the dishes, not having to get out of bed and go to school, or extreme solicitation from father to mother. The birth of the idea — the concept — that if you are having pain, you can avoid doing something you may not want to do or have someone shower you with more affection than usual is easily noted. This concept has nothing special to do with menstrual pain. It has to do with pain, or headache of all types.

Chronic daily headache may certainly, at least at first, garner the sufferer more attention and affection and a release from doing whatever they do not want to do. Unfortunately, the bloom comes off of this rose, but the time it takes to happen may be different for each person. Sooner or later, the spouse, mother, father, or significant other will get tired of the patient constantly being sick and having severe headaches every day. They just want the person to get better, and they start to distance themselves emotionally from the patient. So, what's the patient to do?

Up the ante. Get sicker. Experience more pain. Need to be taken to the hospital emergency room at two in the morning. Need help going to the doctor more often. On a non-conscious level, suffer more to regain the same emotional benefits they had when they first got sick. It is a process of conditioning ... operant conditioning. It is rarely done on a conscious level.

Is this to say that there are not people who take advantage of others, consciously? No, unfortunately. There are a number (very small, thank God) of patients who will tell the doctor their tale of woe and announce that their pain is, on a scale of 0 (no pain) to 10 (the worst pain you could experience without killing yourself), a 12. More importantly, they exhibit no pain behavior, no splinting, no grimacing, no tears, nothing to show they are suffering more pain than they could live with. This is symptom magnification. Or, it may be malingering. It is up to you, the clinician, to determine which it is, and why.

So, what else do we know about the psychology of the chronic headache patient? Well, let's see. There is a major chicken-and-egg problem. We know that depression is secondary to neurochemical changes. We know that chronic headache pain induces changes in, or dysmodulation of, the serotonergic system in the brain. We know that this can induce depression. But, what if the patient was already depressed? Does this cause the headaches? The answer appears to be no, but the onset of chronic headache can markedly exacerbate a pre-existing affective problem. And then they play off of each other — the myofascial pain, the affective changes, and the central nervous system changes — and each seems to make the other worse, or better, if all are dealt with simultaneously.

One thing the insurance adjuster does not want to hear, particularly in a worker's compensation patient, are the words "psychological problem". This opens up an entirely different can of worms and makes them go nuts. After all, they figure, why should getting hit in the head cause a psychological problem? Pain, headache seem reasonable. But depression? Anxiety disorder? Post-traumatic stress disorder? Heavens to Betsy (whoever she is), no way. But, of course, it does happen and it is real.

From a patient's point of view, it is important to perform a thorough evaluation, including imaging studies, if the case indicates they are needed. The patient wants to know (needs to know), first, that what is going on is benign and not associated with a tumor or other pathology, which helps greatly to put their mind at rest; second, that they have a diagnosis, they understand what it is, and it can be treated; and, third, they should not, if they undergo appropriate therapy, get worse.

Fear of the unknown, particularly of the meaning of something unexplained, such as headache, may increase anxiety and depression, which will increase the pain and give the patient more reason to be afraid.

Certain types of assumptions have been agreed upon. That is, in stable, benign pain conditions, patients are more likely to develop pain behaviors which are learned (operant) under environmental control than patients with pain behaviors which are secondary to a pathological process that is unstable.[185]

Fordyce[185] compared these two sources of control: the difference between environmental processes and nociception is, essentially, the difference between operant and reflexive behaviors. For example, if one breaks his or her arm, splinting the arm close to the body by the upper cervical, back, and shoulder muscles can be considered a reflex reaction to pain and a way to protect the injured limb. If the splinting continues after physiological healing has occurred, it is considered a behavioral change secondary to "pleasant" or "good" adaptations to the pain that was there initially. If, for instance, it gets someone off the baseball team, which is something they could not have done before their injury, that learned behavior of avoidance may continue. A possibly silly example, but the point is made.

What a number of clinicians forget is that even "learned behaviors" may have a small (or even large) nidus of real (organic) pain behind them. In the above example of the broken arm, when X-rays reveal that the arm is satisfactorily knit, the cast is removed. Is that really the end of the story? What if the patient had not received physical therapy of some sort to help break down the reflexive muscle spasm in the shoulders and upper back? The patient may continue to have pain behaviors, which are no longer secondary to the broken arm, at least not primarily but secondarily. Then, as we have seen, the changes in the central nervous system neurochemistry occur, and a whole new ball game is being played, even though the arm is healed, which, to an adjuster or physician, may be the only outcome that is desired. The other, secondary problems were not on the agenda, and, because they are not due to a broken arm (the initial problem), they are thought to be pain behavior, or suffering.

The truly important question is the relationship between behavioral outcomes and a patient's chronic headache. What are the outcomes of a patient's reaction to chronic pain and subsequent behaviors? Does his environment — his family or co-workers — make his life easier? Does he get additional emotional support that fulfills a need? Does he no longer have to do something that he doesn't want to do but had to do before developing the pain? These are the important issues: a patient's behaviors and their reinforcements.

It is important to convey to the patient that you are not being judgmental, that you can appreciate his pain, its chronicity and severity. But, at the same time, it is important to explain that certain types of reinforcement can predispose the patient to continued severity and chronicity of their headache problems. Easily done? No way.

In our society, it is thought to be okay to have a physical problem. Having an emotional problem, however, is not okay. It may make the patient feel they look bad to others. It may make them seem weak. Exposing existing emotional problems such as anger or depression may make a patient feel that their pain is being ignored or is thought to be fallacious or somatasized. It is also certainly uncomfortable to disclose closely held feelings which the patient may even feel ashamed of having.

Showing emotions of almost any and all types may be felt by many patients to be "indecent exposure". This concept is important to remember when dealing with these emotions. Making a patient feel ashamed or embarrassed or having them re-live a significant trauma may make them angry enough to leave treatment or develop an exacerbation of their physical symptoms. Many patients have developed a conviction of their illness — they are convinced that their headaches are secondary to a physical problem such as a tumor. They therefore expect to be treated a certain way: with strong medications and an abundance of testing. When these beliefs are refuted, the patient may become convinced that the clinician is obviously wrong. The patient may become very resistant to any form of psychological inquiry, as it goes against his fundamental belief that the problem is entirely physical in nature. To many people, severe pain requires a severe diagnosis, such as a brain tumor; a benign diagnosis again may go against their ingrained feelings.

> **AH HA!** *This is why, when treating a patient with chronic headache who has a significant emotional component to his pain, it may be necessary to give the patient concurrent physical treatment, such as physical therapy for muscle spasm. You will not get the patient to work with you, the clinician, if he thinks that you think the problem is "just in his head". Performing limited physical therapy on these patients concurrently with the psychotherapy grounds their fears by letting them know they are being treated physically, for a physical problem, while the really important treatment is being done in the psychologist's office.*

Many patients may also feel irresponsible or incompetent when told that their headache problems are secondary to stress or anger, things which the patients feel they should be able to control. And there you are, telling them in so many words that they let the stress get to them and it caused their headaches. They may feel angry at the assumption that they could not stop such an "innocuous" problem as stress from getting to them, and they address their anger at, not necessarily to, their physician.

What is stress? It really depends on the patient. If he works in a high-stress job with other people who do not get headaches, he may feel incompetent in that he developed a "stress-related illness" while his co-workers did not. He may take it as a personal attack on his abilities.

There is a cognitive component to stress. This is one readily available place to begin a dialogue with a patient. One definition of stress is that it is a "relationship between the person and the environment that is appraised by the person as taxing or exceeding his or her resources and endangering his or her well-being."[186] The cognitive aspect is the patient's own appraisal of his environment and the interactions he experiences in it. It is true that a specific event may engender a multitude of different responses from participants, from calmness to emotional devastation, so it is not a good idea to compare one person's reaction to another's. It is differences in patients' cognitive thoughts, experiences, and attributions that engender different reactions to the same stimuli. Learning to change beliefs and attributions is helpful to patients who need to learn how to reduce their stress.

Another definition of stress is simpler: "a demand upon energy."[188] Selye defined stress as "the non-specific response of the body to any demand upon it."[189] It should be realized that stress places demands upon all aspects of the human body — neurochemical and physical and physiological. If the initial stress-related arousal levels are ignored, stress-related disease may follow. This may include headache, ulcer, allopecia, or other pathophysiological processes.

It was realized long ago that major life events such as divorce or death of a spouse can have a strong relationship to disease. Of more recent interest is the fact that the more mundane daily stressors, called "daily hassles", may have an even stronger relationship to illness than a so-called major life stressor.[187] This fact, combined with the fact that a patient may not have had any major life changes, may certainly contribute to his insistence that stress has nothing to do with his headaches. These patients may have learned to accommodate to the numerous chronic daily hassles we all live with, but this does not negate their cumulative ill effects.

Change of any type can induce stress, whether the change is perceived by a patient as good or bad. In the phenomenon of the let-down headache, a patient who has endured a stressful period and begins to relax or takes a vacation will get a headache. This may be presumed proof to the patient that the stress did not bring on the headaches, as they had no stress on vacation.

Maladaptive thoughts, or, as one patient put it, "stinking thinking", may also be a contributor to headaches. Patients who set themselves up with unrealistic thoughts such as "if I don't bring home a lot of money every month my wife will leave me" may certainly subject themselves to an inordinate amount of stress, leading to over-activity, poor pacing, and headaches, let-down or otherwise.

The idea of a headache personality was first postulated by Wolff,[190] who described the overly perfectionistic migraine personality. The idea of specific headache personalities, however, has been discarded. Research has been conducted over the years in an attempt to identify any specific psychological pathology that would be pathognemonic to headache patients. It was found that depression was seen more frequently in tension-type headache patients than in patients who had migraine. The "conversion V" found in the first three subcategories of the MMPI (Minnesota Multiphasic Personality Inventory) was thought to be diagnostic for patients with tension-type headache until it was shown that the same "conversion V" was found in patients with chronic low back pain and other chronic, benign pain problems.

Various studies utilizing different psychological tests have been performed, but none succeeded in defining specific pathology attributable to the headache patient.[191–199] It was noted that the levels of daily hassles which induced stress were higher in headache patients.[200,201] Other studies showed that headache patients more typically develop maladaptive coping behaviors in dealing with their headaches.[202,203] Dealing with the issue of "locus of control" may improve the ability to predict which patients may have a better treatment response.[204–206] As no specific psychopathology or personality traits have been identified which would characterize the "typical headache sufferer" individually or by group, extensive psychological testing is not indicated for the "typical headache patient".

Other patients with significant psychological changes — including substance abuse, Waddell's signs on examination, cognitive deficits, personality disorders, or a decline in daily functioning, to name a few — should have a more thorough psychological evaluation performed by a clinical psychologist experienced in the administration and evaluation of the psychological tests used.

The MMPI is frequently used, as is the Millon Clinical Multiaxial Inventory (MCMI), the Behavioral Assessment of Pain (BAP), the Beck Depression Inventory, the Spielberger State/Trait Anxiety Inventory, and the Headache Locus of Control Scales. The Pain Presentation Inventory (PPI) is used more specifically to help determine any aspects of patient reticence to treatment or improvement. Patients with cognitive deficits should have a neuropsychological evaluation by an experienced, specially trained neuropsychologist to determine the presence of traumatically induced cognitive difficulties. Mild traumatic brain injury (MTBI) does not cause post-traumatic headaches, but they are the most common symptom associated with MTBI.

Headache and depression must be ameliorated prior to performing a neuropsychological evaluation. So, the clinician must perform a multidimensional, interdisciplinary evaluation of the chronic headache patient. The headache symptoms must be addressed along with the psychosocial context in which they occur. There is no need, initially, to perform more than a routine psychological screen, as headache patients do not typically present with significant clinical levels of psychopathology. If such psychological problems are revealed during the initial screening tests, then further psychological assessment is needed.

It is important to perform the psychological evaluation on chronic headache patients, because personality disorders, such as a borderline personality disorder, may make treatment more difficult if not dealt with accordingly. The initial assessment may also be important, as it can identify psychological and/or behavioral factors which have a role in maintaining the chronicity of the headache problem.

People are multi-dimensional. To treat a chronic headache patient physically without an understanding of any emotional/behavioral/psychological issues will make the chances of successfully helping the patient's headache problem almost nil. Myogenic nociception, neurochemical dysmodulation, sleep disorders, medication abuse, and a myriad of other physical or medical problems are still associated with the patient's reaction to them. The patient's behaviors, responses to those behaviors or their reinforcement, and the patient's history, experiences, and learned behaviors are equally important. They, and all aspects of the patient taken as a whole person, must be dealt with appropriately to achieve headache amelioration or even a total end to the headache problem.

Various studies have shown another very important fact. At least one third of the female patients (the majority are women) with chronic daily headache have a history of physical or sexual abuse. This is extremely important to identify, as the anger, depression, and non-physical scars may indeed have a relationship to that patient's current problem with chronic headache. Possibly not so amazingly, the headache clinician may be the first medical person to ask about such trauma to a patient who has never before shared the pain and emotional toll the experience has had on her or, less frequently, him. Patients with such experiences who have never dealt appropriately with it may be quite reticent to share this information. The clinician, even if he strongly suspects it, should never bully the patient to get this information. It will come forward if the patient feels safe with the treating clinician/team.

Dealing with the emotional aspects of chronic headache can be more devastating to the patient than dealing with their fears of the etiology of their headaches. It must be done gently, with proper respect for the patient's feelings as well as confidentiality. On the other hand, it may be quite necessary for the psychologist who has obtained the information, whatever it is, to share it with the physician leading the treatment team, as well as, in some cases, other members of the team. For instance, a patient who is afraid of men after being raped, would not be optimally treated by a male physical therapist. A patient who is afraid of male authority figures may need to be dealt with differently than others who are not, particularly if the physician is a male who looks or acts like the object of their fear, i.e., their fathers, their abusers, their husbands, etc.

A good treatment team knows how to implement such changes to enhance patient treatment and effective outcome. If they do not, they will not be able to help the patient and will become, to the patient, another clinician or group of clinicians not able to help in the "impossibly difficult medical odyssey," to quote a patient. It is never easy to deal with all aspects of a patient's physical and psychological condition. It is difficult, many times, to determine what mental or emotional mine fields are present before you wander unknowingly into one.

That is part of the challenge in treating the chronic headache patient. If you cannot enjoy it, at least expect it. Whatever else you do, if you decide to treat the chronic headache patient understand that one clinician, even an expert one, is not able to deal with all of the various aspects of a patient's problems. That is why the most effective treatment is provided by an interdisciplinary headache treatment team. We will discuss that in detail in another chapter, but next we will spend some wood pulp talking about other, specific headache disorders.

chapter nine

Post-traumatic headache

Post-traumatic headache (PTHA) is an extremely common disorder following motor vehicle accidents, slipping and falling, violent altercations, and work-related injuries. It is frequently part of the postconcussive syndrome, which refers to a large number of signs and symptoms that may follow a blow to the head or an acceleration/deceleration injury, which may or may not induce a mild traumatic brain injury (MTBI).

A review article regarding MTBI which details the clinical data as well as clinical evaluation and treatment has recently been published.[207] There are a number of problems involved with this diagnosis that make treatment, even for PTHA, more difficult.

An often-asked question is why people who play various sports for a living, such as football players, wrestlers, boxers, and others, do not have a high incidence of PTHA and/or MTBI. The answer is simple. These people are physically very well conditioned, and when they play they are always prepared and anticipate the possibility of physical trauma. This differentiates them from the vast majority of people who are not even close to being in optimal physical condition who are injured unexpectedly, before they are even aware of the oncoming trauma.

Research has shown that when the head is free, rather than confined, it is more susceptible to acceleration/deceleration injury. As far back as 1941 it was shown in cats that less force was required to produce concussion when the head was free to move compared to when it was fixed, or confined, in place.[208] The concept of "whiplash" (or acceleration/deceleration injury) is important, as it involves a multitude of medical aspects. When an acceleration/deceleration incident occurs (most frequently from a rear-end accident), the physical, or gravitational forces of a massive object such as a car striking another automobile are passed onto the most fragile and movable object not firmly secured in the automobile that was struck: the passenger. Even when the passenger is wearing a seatbelt, the head — essentially a ball at the end of a tether (the neck) — is thrown first forward and then backwards, when the tether can reach no farther and snaps back. If the head is turned at the moment of impact, the rotational forces are also very important to take into account, particularly when a MTBI is found.

There are many folks involved in the insurance aspects of medicine, in addition to the medical and legal aspects, who make a good bit of money by testifying that such physical forces, especially when there was not a great deal of damage to the car, "could in no way cause any organic problems." Typically, these hired guns do not treat patients, which makes them unaware of the realities of the medical challenges found in these patients.

It has been stated that loss of consciousness and/or post-traumatic amnesia must occur if a patient is to develop any medical problems such as MTBI. A more recent definition of MTBI produced by the Brain Injury Interdisciplinary Special Interest Group (BISIG), a part of the American Congress of Rehabilitation Medicine, is far more accurate and unbiased, when one considers the source — experts from multiple medical specialties.[209] It states that a patient with mild traumatic brain injury is a person who has had a traumatically induced physiological disruption of brain function, as manifested by at least one of the following:

- Any period of loss of consciousness
- Any loss of memory for events immediately before or after the accident
- Any alteration in mental state at the time of the accident (e.g., feeling dazed, disoriented, or confused)
- Focal neurological deficit(s) which may or may not be transient

The severity of the injury will not exceed the following limits:

- Loss of consciousness of approximately 30 minutes or less
- An initial Glasgow Coma Scale of 13 to 15 found after 30 minutes
- Post-traumatic amnesia not greater than 24 hours

It is important to note that the definition includes patients with direct head trauma as well as those who suffer an acceleration/deceleration injury without direct head trauma. Loss of consciousness is not a clinical requisite for the diagnosis of MTBI. The symptoms of MTBI may last for varying lengths of time and can consist of persistent physical, emotional, cognitive, and behavioral symptoms which may produce a functional disability. The number of people who experience head trauma of varying degrees is over 2.5 million a year, with the vast majority of them never reaching an emergency room.

The postconcussive syndrome (PCS) may be associated with true MTBI or may occur on a transient basis. The most common medical problems found in the patient with PCS include:

- Post-traumatic headache
- Post-traumatic musculoskeletal pain syndromes
- Vestibular disturbance
- Visual disturbance
- Fatigue

We will not get into, here, the most common cognitive, emotional, and behavioral deficits associated with PCS in patients with MTBI. The pathophysiology of MTBI is nonetheless important in our discussion of post-traumatic headache.

Minor traumatic brain injury may be secondary to one or more of three major pathological features: (1) acceleration/deceleration of the head, (2) skull distortion with resultant pressure gradients intracranially, and (3) cervical spine stretching, which induces myofascial difficulties along with autonomic nervous problems in some patients.[210]

As previously noted, direct head trauma is not necessary in the etiology of MTBI. The speed, magnitude, and direction of the acceleration/deceleration force are the determining factors in regard to the extent and permanence of axonal dysfunction, as it is the inertial force transmitted from sudden deceleration which produces diffuse axonal injury, a major part of the pathophysiology of MTBI.

The existence of diffuse axonal injury (DAI) following an acceleration/deceleration injury (or "whiplash") may be associated with a normal neurological examination. Pathological changes seen in postmortem examination have been found to include DAI, as well as other signs of axonal degeneration.[211–217]

A second major cause of MTBI is significant changes in the post-traumatic neurochemical milieu. Changes have been noted in calcium ions[218] (which can also induce neuronal injury), as well as in the neuroexcitatory neurotransmitters acetylcholine and glutamate. Surges in these neurochemicals after injury contribute to neuronal "burnout" or cell death.[219–223]

Another site of injury at the time of MTBI is the disruption of the blood-brain barrier, which allows further damage to the brain secondary to an influx of circulating excitatory neurotransmitters.[224] Neither CAT scans nor MRIs typically show these pathological deficits in the patient with MTBI secondary to their resolution; these problems are microscopic in nature.

The PCS, in which post-traumatic headache is very common, can be short lived or chronic and disabling, with the possible difference being due to the interaction between the organic and psychological factors.[225] Some feel that the common PCS symptoms (headache, dizziness, irritability) result from emotional stress associated with diminished cognitive performance secondary to MTBI,[226] but there is considerable evidence to suggest that the PCS is primarily a physiological disturbance.[227] Reaction time testing has been used to support a structural, organic etiology for the PCS.[228]

It is felt by this author and others that the term "postconcussive syndrome" should encompass the non-neurological/neurocognitive and neurophysiological deficits, leaving the term PCS to mean the post-traumatic signs and symptoms for the other non-cerebral organ systems which may be affected.

Immediately after MTBI, the majority of patients have complaints attributable to several different organ systems. One clinician[229] has identified these complaints as being PCS. He notes that PCS that can lead to brain injury can also cause injury to the head, the neck ("whiplash" and soft tissue damage), the vestibular system, and psychological functioning. The initial complaints of deficits in cognition and sleep disorder are secondary to neuronal injury, while the headache may be secondary to cervical injury, neuronal injury, or a combination of the two; neck pain, secondary to soft tissue problems; dizziness, secondary to peripheral vestibular dysfunction, soft tissue, or cervical injury; and anxiety, moodiness, and irritability, secondary to neurological injury, pain, and/or psychological factors.

After one year, 85 to 90% of patients are felt to be "recovered" but are still symptomatic, leaving, therefore, 10 to 15% of patients who not only are "not recovered" and but are still very symptomatic.[230,231] Existing literature shows persistence of symptoms far longer than the magical 3- to 6-month period which many clinicians state is as long as it should take for spontaneous healing to occur. The literature indicates that the symptoms and deficits following MTBI, including headache, may last for 6 to 12 months and even longer.[232–238]

One survey showed that rehabilitation specialists noted 21% of patients experienced PCS symptoms 2 to 6 months after initial injury.[239] Another survey found that 25% of patients reported continued sequelae from their injury. The patients with sequelae after one year were found to have reported the most symptoms one week after initial injury.[240]

Persistent postconcussive syndrome (PPCS) was noted to be found in patients who, after one year, continue to complain of symptoms commonly seen in acute PCS, including headache. They were also noted to have prominent emotional symptoms including irritability, depression, nervousness, discouragement, and anger.[241] Other authors noted that pain severity post-injury was a predictor of the development of the PPCS.[241–243] Data also suggest a greater frequency of anxiety and depression months after initial injury.[244]

Chronic headache and pain are fairly universal accompaniments of PPCS. It is also noted that patients with chronic headache not associated with MTBI or the PPCS have many of the same complaints, including fatigue, depression, sleep disorder, and even dizziness, as well as problems with memory and concentration. It has also been noted that psychological factors may aggravate these headaches.

The factors of pain and headache, especially the chronic post-traumatic tension-type headache, have been extensively described.[84,117,245,246] The pathophysiology was described earlier (Chapter 6) as being a combination of myofascial nociception and affective changes (which develop over time secondary to the headache pain and neurochemical changes) which induce significant changes in the neurochemistry of the central nervous system. These changes, which include neuronal exhaustion and the "empty neuron syndrome", are associated with significant changes in the serotonergic, noradrenergic, and endogenous opiate neurotransmitter systems. These central nervous system neurochemical changes become the primary etiology of the continued headache (see Figure 1 in Chapter 7).

In patients with chronic post-traumatic tension-type headache associated with MTBI, the above problems exist in concert with the other neurophysiological and neurochemical problems noted earlier in this chapter. Aside from diffuse axonal injury, which may interfere with higher cortical functions, as well as perception, there are the post-traumatic neurochemical problems of excitotoxic cell injury and death and the opening of the blood-brain barrier (for 8 to 12 hours) immediately post-injury, which can also lead to an influx of excitotoxic neurochemicals that can also lead to cell death.

Bottom line is that the neurochemical factors leading to the perpetuation of the tension-type headaches appear to be further and more complexly involved than those found in the form of chronic tension-type headache not associated with MTBI. Treatment is again found to be most appropriately and cost-effectively performed in an interdisciplinary headache rehabilitation program. Tricyclic medications, GABAnergic medications, and NSAIDs are appropriate.

There are several caveats. First, if MTBI is suspected (with associated diminution of cognitive abilities), then narcotics, dilantin, barbiturates, and early forms of benzodiazepines should not be used, as they will further diminish cognitive ability. Second, one should not attempt to test for cognitive abilities in the presence of headache pain and depression. They must be ameliorated prior to neuropsychological testing. Third, is an ...

> **AH HA!** *Patients with minor traumatic brain injury who also complain of headache do not appear to perceive their headache pain accurately. They know they have it. On a scale of 0 (no pain) to 10 (pain so severe you could not tolerate it for a moment or two), individual patients, when first seen, will give you a high number, e.g. 7 to 10, which is correlated to pathophysiological myofascial findings, including decreased cervical range of motion, muscle spasm, active trigger points, and more. As you treat them, you will see them regain appropriate physical functioning: normal cervical range of motion, obliteration of spasm and trigger points, etc., with a marked associated improvement of function. The patients will have a brighter affect, smile, have no pain behaviors, and resume doing the physical things they enjoy. Yet, when asked, they will continue to state that their headache pain is*

at the same level of 7 to 10 as when they were first seen. Whether they are perseverating or are just unable to give an accurate subjective pain level, their stated pain levels do not change very much. Therefore, you must evaluate them on improvements in function, not by self-reported decrements in headache pain levels.

There are other types of headache secondary to head trauma or acceleration/deceleration injury. Migraine (with and without aura) has been seen in patients who may be susceptible to migraine but who have never had one before head trauma.[247–249] Trauma may induce the first migraine attack in a susceptible patient or increase the frequency and possibly the severity of pre-existing migraine. The etiology of these changes may be secondary to neuronal and axonal abnormalities secondary to trauma. Treatment is typically with beta-blockers such as propranolol. The use of valproic acid is also useful. Cluster headache has been seen secondary to head trauma, again probably secondary to neuronal and axonal injury. Treatment is the same as noted in the cluster headache chapter.

After soft tissue injury of the scalp or face, there may occur an entrapment of a sensory nerve, or the sensory nerve may have been cut during the trauma via laceration. The entrapment may also occur during suturing of a laceration. Such entrapments cause nerve, or neuropathic, pain. This is easily differentiated from the other primary headache types. The pain is constant, burning, and relegated to the sensory distribution of the affected nerve. Typically the best treatment is anticonvulsant medications such as carbamazepine. In some cases, neurolytic procedures such as radiofrequency coagulation or cryo-ablation may be necessary. Both are good procedures but have varying durations of benefit, typically 6 to 12 months or so.

A patient may have any or all of the above post-traumatic headache or pain problems. Diagnosis is obviously important. It is frequently a good idea to utilize both a tricyclic and beta-blocker (or other migraine prophylactic medication) together if you are unsure of the presence of both tension-type and vascular headache.

Injuries may also occur to the cervical spine, to the superficial and deep structures of the neck: muscle, ligaments, bone, discs, or nerve roots. Cervical pain, from trigger points in spasmed muscle as well as from cervical joint dysfunction, may be referred to the head. Pain may be sub-occipital with lancinating, electrical-like shooting pain, secondary to involvement of the occipital neurovascular bundle (the occipital nerve, artery, and vein), secondary to prolonged muscle contraction or excessive vascular dilatation impinging on the greater occipital nerve of Arnold. The pain is known as occipital neuralgia and is always in the C_2 region at the back of the head. Indomethacin is the best treatment for this. Steroidal injections may also be needed. Pre-existing arthritis or even discogenic disease may also be exacerbated by the initial trauma.

As usual, psychological factors should be assessed in patients with post-traumatic headache syndrome, particularly if they have had the problem for 2 to 3 months or more. Both a patient's reaction to the injury as well as problems produced by organic injury may be involved, and trying to tease out how much of which problem exists is probably not worth your time. Both problems are typically involved. Your problem is in treating the depression and/or anxiety in conjunction with the headache diathesis. Various studies show that headaches that are going to remit spontaneously will do so within several months. Patients' headaches that will stop will have done so in 4 years! This study[250] did not look at treatment.

The major problems facing patients and their treating physician(s) are the questions of medicolegal disability secondary to the post-traumatic headache syndrome with or without the question of MTBI (which *always* makes life more difficult). With patients whose injuries have involved a skull fracture, intracranial bleeding, or severe lacerations and whose gray matter is leaking from their ears, there *may* not be a problem in regard to disability. Unfortunately, even with these aspects in the history, insurance problems do exist, beginning with getting approval to treat.

Some insurance companies have taken the tack that MTBI does not exist. Period. They will fight tooth and nail, with a heck of a lot of money backing them up, to prove it. They will prevent clinicians from even getting involved with treating these patients by refusing to pay them for treatment. It does not matter how devastating the patient's symptoms are; the patient will still face a tough, unjustifiable legal battle just to get treatment approved, never mind the question of disability compensation.

Hired guns exist. These are people with some medical background who do not treat patients, but who testify that, in their august opinions and by looking at the mode of injury, the patients could not have sustained any post-traumatic injury, physical or cognitive. When you treat these patients, you have to be prepared to deal with these folk.

On the other hand, the fact that they spend their entire lives as hired guns — evaluating patients and testifying in trial against the diagnoses given them by their treating physicians — may begin to be detrimental to them. In the state of Colorado, physicians who wish to do independent medical examinations for insurance companies now have to prove that they actually treat patients and that they do these insurance examinations less than 50% of their practice time. Just a "heads up"; if you have not run into this sham, you probably will in the future.

It is a most interesting phenomenon that the vast majority of patients with the postconcussive syndrome present the same way. Either they all got together and planned their symptoms, which means they are very knowledgeable of the medical literature, *or* they are for real and expressing the same symptoms from the same causation (head trauma or acceleration/deceleration injury). This is just like patients with chicken pox who initially all present, clinically, in about the same way.

Then, of course, there is the M word — malingering. This is associated with the idea that settlement of litigation is all that is needed to put a stop to the symptoms of the post-traumatic syndrome. This is also a favorite theme of the insurance companies. True malingering is almost as rare as hens' teeth. Studies have demonstrated that legal settlement has nothing to do with the patients' symptoms ending nor encouraging them to return to work.[251–254]

Chronic post-traumatic headache, along with the other aspects of the postconcussive syndrome (again, we are not talking here about MTBI), are extremely common after head trauma as well as an acceleration/deceleration injury ("whiplash"). The patients with these problems are amazingly consistent in their descriptions of their symptoms and sequelae. This consistency is strong evidence that their problems are organic in nature and produced by the trauma. Most patients with post-traumatic headache will get better if they are afforded appropriate medical treatment. About 15 to 20% will have prolonged difficulties. Appropriate treatment may decrease this percentage. If the patient can get it.

Well, another sacred cow slaughtered. There is such a thing as post-traumatic headache, and it is treatable. Boy, imagine that. Now, just for the sake of something different, let's look at orofacial pain.

chapter ten

Orofacial pain

Well, we have done the primary headache disorders. Congratulations! Now we are going to move onto the less frequent headache/facial pain problems. Remember, organic causes of headache account for about one half of one percent of all headache problems. They are rare, but you certainly do not want to miss them. Because the medicine behind some of the following entities can be rigorous, I will try not to go into as much detail as found in the past chapters.

Let's start inside the mouth, with some common etiologies of intra-oral pain, as well as some that are not so common:

- Infection, abscess
- Viral infection (herpetic)
- Inflammation (pulpitis)
- Trauma
- Bruxism
- Referred myofascial pain
- Atrophic candidiasis
- Ulcerative mucositis (includes Bechet's syndrome)
- Benign mucus membrane pemphigoid (an erosive/desquamative disorder)
- Erythema multiforme

As you know, to evaluate pulpal pain the use of electovitalometers, thermal tests, and periodontal ligament diagnostic anesthetic blocks may supplement clinical and radiological examinations. If you know your anatomy, specifically the places to which pain from specific trigger points can radiate, you know that trigger point pain can radiate to the normal teeth as well as from the mouth to the temporomandibular (TM) joint. If that is suspected, put on a glove and palpate the lateral pterygoid muscle. If it is extremely tender, use a tuberculin syringe to inject about .5 cc of lidocaine without epinephrine. Other myalgic pain syndromes may originate in the medial pterygoid, the buccinator, the mylohyoid, the omohyoid muscle, and the short and long head of the temporal muscle tendons.

Ligamentous pain syndromes can include hyoid bone syndrome, Eagle's syndrome (stylohyoid ligament insertion tendinitis), stylomandibular and sphenomandibular ligamentous pain, and capsular ligament pain. These craniomandibular pain syndromes may be best diagnosed and dealt with by a dentist or oral surgeon who has experience in the differential diagnosis of these problems, as well as the ability to perform a differential neural blockade.

Of course, first you usually have to do your typically excellent history and physical examination/neurological examination, with or without appropriate lab studies, and possibly a psychological evaluation, before you can know that you should send the patient out for referral ... unless the history is specific enough.

There are a number of pertinent neuralgic and neuritic pain syndromes which affect the face. Post-herpetic neuralgia is secondary to herpes zoster viral infection. It follows the distribution of the involved trigeminal nerve division. It may be associated with odontalgia. It may also produce excessive scarring and fibrosis at nerve terminals. There is a peripheral loss of afferent inhibition — specifically, the loss of large-diameter sensory nerves such as the A-delta nerves. It may be difficult to control the pain. Treatment should start early with burst steroids. Followup treatment may include capsaicin and anticonvulsants, with carbamazepine being the drug of choice.[255–258]

Glossopharyngeal neuralgia is an electrical-like pain in the ear or throat, with an associated trigger in the throat. The anterior, inferior cerebellar artery usually is compressing the rootlets of cranial nerves IX and X, and neurosurgical decompression is needed. It may also be associated with laryngeal carcinoma; these patients may also have trigeminal neuralgia.[259]

Carotidynia is an episodic, throbbing, deep, dull neck pain with occasional neck swelling. There are two types. One is associated with migraine and is treated with vasoactive medications. The other is associated with arthritis and is treated with NSAIDs or corticosteroids. At least one of the following is noted to overlay the carotid artery: tenderness, swelling, or increased pulsations. Laboratory investigations do not reveal any structural abnormality. The pain over the neck may project to the ipsilateral side of the head. It is self limiting, usually less than 2 weeks. This diagnosis, in spite of having an International Headache Society diagnostic code, is not felt to be a validated entity. Carotidynia is thought by many to be nothing more than a unilateral neck pain associated with local tenderness that can be secondary to a number of vascular and nonvascular etiologies (including fibromuscular dysplasia, giant cell arteritis, lymphadenitis, local aphtous ulcers, and malignant infiltration).[260–266]

The neck-tongue syndrome is an uncommon problem characterized by attacks of occipital pain precipitated by sudden rotation of the head and associated with a subjective sensation of numbness in the ipsilateral side of the tongue. It is probably secondary to the C_2 nerve being compressed by the lateral atlantoaxial joint. Treatment may be via immobilization by a soft collar. In some cases, atlantoaxial fusion or resection of the C_2 spinal nerves has been performed.[267–271]

Painful ophthalmoplegia may be secondary to a variety of problems, including superior orbital fissure syndrome, orbital apex syndrome, cavernous sinus syndrome, parasellar syndrome, and Tolosa-Hunt syndrome. It is unilateral, with an associated paralysis of one or more cranial nerves: III, IV, or VI. There is an associated parasympathoplegia or sympathoplegia of the eye. There is no structural lesion, and granulomatous tissue may be seen on MRI. While there may be a chronic inflammatory process involving the carotid sinus, carotid artery, and orbit, no known etiology is recognized. It responds to steroid therapy. A Horner's syndrome may be present.[272–276]

Ramsey Hunt syndrome is secondary to a herpes zoster infection of the sensory and motor branches of cranial nerve VII and, occasionally, VIII. It can cause deafness, vertigo, and facial paralysis. Herpetic lesions can be found in the ear and on the anterior tongue and soft palate. Treatment includes analgesics.

Raeder's syndrome consists of severe unilateral frontal headache followed by ipsilateral Horner's syndrome. It usually affects men in the fifth decade and is secondary to a disorder of the pericarotid sympathetic plexus in the cavernous sinus.[277,278]

Post-traumatic neuralgia (also known as anesthesia dolorosa, as well as central pain and thalamic pain) is characterized by painful anesthesia or dysesthesia often related to surgical trauma of the trigeminal ganglion, especially after the performance of rhizotomy or thermocoagulation for the treatment of idiopathic trigeminal neuralgia or after specific vascular lesions of the central trigeminal pathways. It is limited to the distribution of one or more divisions of the trigeminal nerve. Sensation to pin prick is diminished over the affected area. This pain syndrome is probably one of the most difficult to treat. Narcotics and other analgesics do not help a great deal. Further surgery typically is not helpful for more than a short period. Electrical stimulation of the gasserian ganglion may be effective. Tricyclic antidepressants or stellate ganglion blocks may be helpful. Repeated anesthetic blocks done early may be helpful to the long-term outcome. The psychological and behavioral treatment of the patient is important.[279–287]

Trigeminal neuralgia is the best known of the facial neuralgias. It is associated with electrical-like facial pain associated with intra- and extraoral triggers. Not uncommonly, patients may be seen with only one side of their face shaved, or make-up on only one side of their face, as they will not want to do anything to arouse a trigger to their pain. It may be associated with ipsilateral demyelinated microneuromas in the trigeminal rootlets or with vascular compression of the rootlets of the trigeminal nerve at the entrance zone to the pons. Neurosurgical decompression, rhizotomy of the mandibular division, radiofrequency lesions of the affected divisions, or retrogasserian glycerol injection should follow an adequate trial of anticonvulsants (carbamazepine, valproic acid) and GABAnergic medications (baclofen, clonazepam).[288–299] It must be realized that treatment with anticonvulsants for neuralgic or neuropathic pain is different than treatment for seizures. The typical dose of carbamazepine is 200 mg three times a day for seizures. For nerve-related pain, the dosage may need to go up to 1400 to 1800 mg a day. Extreme care must be taken to prevent aplastic anemia and hepatic dysfunction.

There is another entity called "pre-trigeminal neuralgia" which may be easily misdiagnosed. It has a toothache-like presentation. The pain is longer lasting and is often dull or aching in quality.[300,301] Pre-trigeminal neuralgia must be differentiated from small tumors inducing pain, atypical odontalgia or facial pain, facial or "lower half" migraine, toothache of pulpal origin, sinusitis, and temporomandibular joint (TMJ) dysfunction. It is important to differentiate among trigeminal neuralgia, pre-trigeminal neuralgia, and dental pain to avoid unnecessary tooth extraction.[302,303]

Atypical facial pain is characterized by persistent facial pain that does not have the characteristics of the cranial neuralgias and is not associated with physical signs or a demonstrable organic lesion. The pain is present daily and is constant. It is confined at the onset to a limited area on one side of the face, but it may spread to the upper or lower jaws or to a wider area of the face or neck. The pain is deep, poorly localized, and not associated with sensory loss or other physical signs. Laboratory investigations are negative. The pain is more common in women than men. Analgesics and nerve blocks do not help. Evidence exists that these patients have significant psychopathology. Tricyclic antidepressants and psychotherapy may be helpful.[304–308]

Burning tongue and mouth may be related to hormonal status, chronic depression, denture irritation, or vitamin B deficiency. Atypical odontalgia or neurovascular odontalgia may be possible variants of cluster headache. A painful toothache with no local pathological process in or around the tooth or gums may be secondary to referred pain from myofascial trigger points.

There are other benign vascular forms of headache with which you should be familiar. These include:

- Migrainous-type cephalalgia in post-endarterectory patients, which is transient and benign
- Benign orgasmic headache, of which there are three types with two being indomethacin responsive
- Benign exertional headache, also indomethacin responsive
- Migrainous-type headache or aura seen with lupus cerebral vasculitis
- Ice-pick headache (ophthalmodynia periodica), a unilateral, jabbing pain at the temple or orbit; benign
- Ice cream headache, perhaps more common in migraineurs and resulting from sudden cooling of the oral pharynx and blood in the internal carotid artery; essentially a trigeminal nerve effect

Temporomandibular joint disorders may cause headache which disappears after successful treatment of the disorder. Functional disorders and pain in the anatomic region of the TMJ and associated musculature are referred to as temporomandibular disorders (TMDs). Using the American Academy of Orofacial Pain classification system,[309] which conforms to the International Headache Society classification, it is estimated that of the 70% of patients with signs of TMD only 5% will require treatment and even fewer will complain of headache.

The TMJ is a diarthroidial synovial joint which is characterized as having two compartments separated by fibrous disks. The joint movements are both rotational as well as translational. The first 25 mm of mouth opening involve the rotation of the condyle within the fossa. The second 25 mm involve translation of the disk condyle complex along the articular eminence. TMDs are classified as either joint-related problems (arthrogenous) or muscle disorders (myogenous). They may occur together or individually. Inflammation within the joint may induce TMJ pain, which is complicated by dysfunctions of the intracapsular components, the ligaments, and disk. The most frequent cause of TMJ pain and related headache is myofascial. On examination, masticatory muscle tenderness is common. Other etiological factors for TMD-associated headache include bruxism, trauma, occlusal interferences, and emotional stressors.[310–313]

Inflammation of the TMJ is mostly associated with degenerative changes seen on imaging studies. Both rheumatoid and psoriatic arthritis can affect the TMJ. Inflammation of the TMJ may also occur in conjunction with internal derangements or incoordinations of disk condyle and temporal bone. Joint noise heard with movement may be secondary to anatomic changes to any of the articulating surfaces secondary to changes from micro- or macrotraumas. Crepitation may also be noted when the disk is displaced, typically anteriorly and laterally. When this occurs, there is rotation of the condyle up to 25 mm of interincisal opening, and at this point the patient may experience "catching" secondary to binding of the disk against the eminence. The jaw will then translate after manipulation or movement of the mandible, which will cause a clicking or popping noise as the condyle moves under the disk. This describes the anterior displacement of the disk with reduction. There is usually associated intracapsular inflammation.

The diagnostic criteria of TMD includes at least two of the following: (1) pain of the jaw precipitated by movement and/or clenching, (2) decreased range of movement, (3) noise during joint movements, and (4) tenderness of the joint capsule. These findings are associated with a positive X-ray and/or isotope scintigraphic findings. The pain is mild to moderate and is located in the TMJ and/or radiates from there.

Pain localized in the muscles of mastication is the most frequent presenting symptom, along with localizations in the preauricular region or the TMJ itself. The pain is increased by jaw function. Other characteristics are decreased or asymmetrical jaw movement or locking on opening.

Headache is commonly associated with complaints of TMDs. The association of TMDs and headache is thought to be directly related to the pathology of the TMJ or, more commonly, to myofascial problems.[314–316]

Management is typically with physical medicine approaches. The use of an appliance may be justified by TMJ derangement. NSAIDs are useful, as are small doses of tricyclic antidepressants.

One problem is that in the outcome studies of headache related to TMD there are various ways of assessing pain reduction. The generalization has been made that if headache is decreased by treatment of TMD, then the etiology of the pain is the TMD. Unfortunately, few ever comment on the problem of central nervous system neurochemical dysmodulation or even behavioral factors, making the outcome studies poor and the conclusions possibly specious.[314,316–318]

Well, that is the general story about orofacial pain and the like. Now, to make things even more interesting, let us look at other, organic causes of headache.

chapter eleven

Organic causes of headache

One of the biggest challenges in the treatment of headache is diagnosis. As mentioned previously, patients with organic causes of headache are approximately one half of one percent, obviously a relatively small number. The problem is that these patients have the most to lose if you do not diagnose the etiology of their headache correctly. The treatment of headache in these patients lies in treating the underlying pathology, as you are not dealing with one of the previously discussed primary headache disorders. Briefly, the most typical organic causes of headache include:

- Cerebrovascular dilatation
  - Pyrexia and infection
  - Prostaglandins A and E
- Cerebral hypoxia
  - Anemia
  - Myelophthesic disease
  - Toxic hemoglobinopathies
  - Circulatory failure
  - Polycythemia
  - High-altitude headache
- Hypercapnea syndromes
  - Severe scoliosis
  - Chronic obstructive pulmonary disease
  - Pickwickian syndrome
  - Sleep apnea syndrome
  - Chronic CO_2 poisoning
- Traction of intracranial structures
  - Tumor
  - Abcess
  - Hematoma
  - Hydrocephalus

  - Hypertensive encephalopathy
  - Eclampsia
  - Benign intracranial hypertension (pseudotumor cerebri)
  - Post-lumbar puncture
- Endocrine abnormalities
  - Hypo- and hyperthyroidism
  - Cushing's syndrome
  - Addison's disease
- Hypocalcemia
- Cerebral hypoglycemia
- Collagen vascular disease
  - Systemic lupus erythematosus
  - Rheumatoid
  - Polymyalgia rheumatica
  - Scleroderma
- Hemodynamic changes
  - Essential hypertension
  - Exertion
  - Acute pressor reaction
    - Mao inhibitors
    - Sexual intercourse
    - Pheochromocytoma
  - Post-ictal headache
- Drug ingestion and toxicity
  - Nitrates, nitrites
  - Alcohol
  - Toxic levels of lead, benzene, carbon tetrachloride, organophosphates
  - Drug withdrawal
    - Simple and narcotic analgesics taken daily or QOD for more than 1 to 2 weeks
    - Ergots
    - Amphetamines
    - Cocaine
    - Phenothiazines
    - Caffeine
- Cerebrovascular disease
  - Acute subarachnoid hemorrhage
  - Arteriovenous malformations
  - Aneurysms
  - Cerebral venous thrombosis
  - Transient ischemic attack (TIA)
  - Cerebrovascular accident (CVA)
  - S/P carotid endarterectory

As each of these topics is worthy of a book, I will undertake to explore only a small number of them in some detail. Some, of course, are self-explanatory.

Infection

The headache secondary to noncephalic infections typically occurs with fever. Pyrogens can cause increases in arachidonic acid metabolites which include prostaglandins, prostacyclin, and thromboxane. Prostaglandin E_2 (PGE_2) appears to act on the hypothalamus and can initiate fever independent of endogenous pyrogens. In fact, PGE_2 appears to have vasoactive properties and may be implicated, at least indirectly, in the vascular component of such headache.

The International Headache Society's diagnostic criteria for headache associated with noncephalic infection[12] include: symptoms and/or signs of noncephalic infection, laboratory diagnosis of systemic or focal non-cephalic infection, headache as a new symptom or of a new type occurring concomitantly with infection, or headache which disappears less than 1 month after successful treatment or spontaneous remission of the infection.

There is no specific headache type associated with noncephalic infection. It is typically bilateral and diffuse, with pain of variable intensity, described as steady, throbbing, or pulsating, and can be made more intense by movement of the head.

Migraine, cluster, and tension-type headache may be induced by noncephalic infections, secondary to fever, in patients who have a history of these headache diatheses. Interestingly, an association between cluster headache and herpes simplex has been noted.[319]

Sinusitis may induce headache, particularly if the ethmoid and maxillary sinuses are affected. Sphenoid sinusitis may also induce headache, but this diagnosis is more difficult to make. This headache is typically short lived, frequently retro-orbital in location. These headaches may be increased by straining or bending.

Cephalic infections may be life threatening. Meningitis of any type requires quick diagnosis and treatment. The most common bacterial causes in the adult include *Neisseria meningitidis*, *Haemophilus influenzae*, and *Streptococcus pneumoniae*.[320] Aside from generalized headache or suboccipital headache, other classical signs include fever, nuchal rigidity, and altered levels of consciousness. Diagnosis involves an abnormal cerebral spinal fluid examination, typically showing increased protein and decreased glucose, polymorphonuclear pleiocytosis, and confirmation of the pathogen. Meningitis may occur as a result of viruses, mycobacteria, fungi, and parasites. Mollaret's meningitis, or recurrent episodes of viral or "aseptic" meningitis, may be associated with headache and is relatively rare. It may be associated with other neurological signs and symptoms, as well.

Cerebral abscess may be chronic, without manifestation of headache early in the disease process. The associated headache is unrelenting and dull. Treatment, following a cerebral CAT scan or MRI, includes antibiotic therapy and surgical drainage.

Viral encephalitis is also an extremely serious neurological disorder. The two most common causes are herpes simplex and the rabies virus, although post-influenza viral encephalitis has also been noted. The cerebral spinal fluid examination may be normal or show increased cells and protein levels. Acyclovir may be useful in the treatment of the herpes simplex form of encephalitis.

Headache may also be seen secondary to underlying infection with the human immunodeficiency virus (HIV). Patients with AIDS may develop multiple neurological problems, including aseptic meningitis and subacute encephalitis. In an AIDS patient with new onset of headache, cryptococcal meningitis should be ruled out.

Endocrine disorders

Endocrine disorders which can cause headache, typically secondary to vasodilation, include hypoglycemia, hypothyroidism, adrenal insufficiency, and hyperthyroidism. Hyperparathyroidism may induce headache secondary to hypercalcemia or low levels of magnesium.

Collagen vascular disorders

Collagen vascular diseases may also be associated with headache. One of the most frequent associations is seen in patients with systemic lupus erythmatosis.[321] Other diseases in this particular family include polyarteritis nodosa, Wegener's granulomatosis, and scleroderma. Temporal arteritis (giant cell arteritis) is secondary to giant cell infiltration into the walls of the temporal artery, as well as other arteries. The headache, while it may be localized to the visibly enlarged temporal artery, may occur anywhere on the head. The treatment of headache secondary to all of these disorders is typically with corticosteroids, as well as other immunosuppressive agents. The headache associated with the collagen vascular diseases is typically relentless and throbbing. It is important to rule out a central nervous system vasculitis, which may also affect other organ systems. Magnetic resonance angiography (MRA) as well as cerebral angiography may be required to make the diagnosis, which is fairly difficult to make.

Various etiologies

Headache may be seen in association with angina pectoris, and benign exertional headache may be a result of coronary artery disease.[322] Headache may also be associated with significant aortic insufficiency. Hypoxia and hypercarbia, both of which induce cerebral vasodilation with an increased cerebral blood flow, are associated with headache that is typically nocturnal and seen upon awakening. High-altitude headache is also associated with hypoxia. These headaches, as are those seen in obstructive sleep apnea, are typically intense and throbbing. Patients with high-altitude headache may be helped with acetazolamide or dexamethasone, 4 mg every 6 hours beginning at the onset of symptoms. Headache may also be associated with hemodialysis secondary to large water and electrolyte shifts.

As noted in the chapter on migraine, various substances may induce this primary headache disorder, including licorice, nitrates, nitrites (hot dog headache), alcohol, chocolate, caffeine, monosodium glutamate (Chinese restaurant syndrome), tyramine, pesticides, and heavy metal poisoning. Tension-type or combination headache (tension-type with secondary vascular features) may be seen.

Headaches secondary to arterial hypertension may be seen in patients whose diastolic blood pressure ranges from 120 to 140 mm of mercury. These headaches are usually noted in the morning upon awakening, are mild to moderate in severity, and are typically bi-occipital. They may resolve as the patient becomes mobile and ambulates. Prompt attention should be paid to such headache, with hospitalization, if necessary, and use of parenteral antihypertensives until the blood pressure is placed under control. Treatment is then transferred to oral agents.

Pheochromocytoma may induce severe, paroxysmal headache associated with excess catecholamine production and secondary sudden increases in blood pressure. The same form of acute pressor reaction can be seen in patients who mix a monoamino oxidase (MAO) inhibitor medication with tyramine. Sympathomimetic medications such as dextroamphetamine and pseudoephedrine may cause headache.

Cerebrovascular disease

Hemorrhagic cerebrovascular headache may be associated with "warning" headaches secondary to minor leakage of blood from an aneurysm or arteriovascular malformation. These warning headaches are sudden, unilateral, or occipital and can occur several times prior to the major rupture, which causes a "thunder-clap headache", the worst headache in a patient's life, which is frequently associated with gradual or faster loss of consciousness. The warning headaches have been known to occur between 1 day and almost 3 months prior to the major rupture. The headache is secondary to an abrupt rise in intracranial pressure, the direct irritant effects of blood on nerves, and the stimulation of vascular nerves associated with the ruptured vessels or aneurysm.

While the incidence of headache associated with ischemic stroke is between 27 and 30%, its pathophysiology is not well understood.[323] The headache may occur before or at the onset of an ischemic vascular event. Events secondary to the carotid circulation typically cause frontal headache, while occipital headache is seen in basilar-vertebral artery strokes.[324] Headache may also be associated with transient ischemic attacks (TIAs).

Patients with migraine with aura may develop a "migrainous stroke" secondary to significant vasoconstriction during the aura phase of the migraine. The question of this occurring in increased numbers in migrainous women who take estrogenic birth control pills who also smoke is still under debate. Pseudotumor cerebri (benign intracranial hypertension), epilepsy, "postendarterectomy hemicrania", and multiple sclerosis are other neuropathological problems associated with headache.

Cervical spondylosis

The major identifiable cervical problem inducing headache is cervical spondylosis, with reports indicating that headache is associated in 13 to 80% of patients,[325] a rather wide range to be sure, indicative of questionable study techniques.

Space-occupying lesions

The majority of patients who develop headache for the first time are usually frightened about the possibility of a brain tumor. The headache secondary to brain tumors is called a traction headache, as pain-sensitive intracranial structures are involved, secondary to local traction on these areas occurring by the tumor mass itself or distant traction occurring by mass effect or hydrocephalus. Increased intracranial pressure by itself is not reliably associated with headache.[326] This is true in many cases; however, pseudotumor cerebri patients frequently can have headache.

One classical study[327] showed that stimulating different parts of the skull referred pain. Stimulation of the superior surface of the tentorium referred pain to the ipsilateral forehead and eye. Stimulation of the pain-sensitive structures in the posterior fossa referred pain to the ipsilateral ear (through the recurrent meningeal branch of the vagus nerve) and the lower occipital and upper cervical regions (via the three upper cervical nerve roots). Pain from the dura has poor localizing value.

The classical brain tumor headache may be severe, worse in the morning and exacerbated with Valsalva maneuvers, with associated nausea and vomiting. Frequently, the headache is less severe and similar to tension-type headache. It is associated with focal neurological lesions or increased intracranial pressure (increasing nausea and vomiting) and is more intractable to treatment. It is progressive.

Headache symptoms from supratentorial headaches are much more benign in nature when compared to those in the infratentorial regions or tumors with associated increased intracranial pressure. Literature indicates a possible association between benign cough and benign exertional headache and the presence of tumor.[328,329] Treatment involves steroids to decrease edema and surgical mass reduction, to whatever degree possible.

The benign headaches: cough, exertional, and post-coital

The three primary types of benign headaches are noted to be very controllable with indomethacin. Benign cough headache is described as headache precipitated by coughing, in the absence of intracranial pathology. The International Headache Society criteria[12] include bilateral headache of sudden onset, lasting less than one minute and precipitated by coughing; it may be prevented by not coughing and may be diagnosed after structural lesions such as posterior fossa tumors have been excluded by neuroimaging. Treatment is with indomethacin, 50 mg three times a day. Of course, you must rule out the presence of an Arnold-Chiari malformation or other lesion inducing an obstruction of cerebral spinal fluid pathways or displacing cerebral structures to assure the diagnosis of benign cough headache.

Benign exertional headache is one precipitated by any form of exercise, apparently secondary to arterial dilatation. Its diagnostic criteria[12] include a headache that is specifically brought on by physical exercise; it is bilateral and throbbing in nature at onset and may develop migrainous features in patients susceptible to migraine. The headache lasts from 5 minutes to 24 hours and are avoided by not participating in excessive exertion, especially in hot weather or at high altitudes. They are not associated with any form of systemic or intracranial pathology. Again, indomethacin is the treatment of choice, 50 mg three times a day, or a 75-mg sustained release form taken 2 hours before exercise.

Headache associated with sexual activity (benign sex headache) may be brought on by masturbation or coitus, typically beginning as a dull bilateral ache while sexual excitement increases and becoming markedly intense at orgasm, in the absence of any intracranial disorder. There are three types of post-orgasmic cephalalgia. The first, the dull type, is noted to be a dull ache in the head and neck which increases in severity as sexual excitement increases. It is felt that muscle contraction appears to be a major feature of this headache. The second type, the explosive type, occurs with a sudden severe or explosive headache at orgasm. This headache may be occipital or generalized, is often throbbing, and may be associated with palpitations. It may be secondary to an acute pressor response to increases in blood pressure at the time of orgasm.

Treatment of the first type may include muscle relaxation training, as well as the use of 50 or 75 mg of indomethacin taken an hour or two before attempting coitus. The same treatment (indomethacin) has been noted by this author and others to be effective for the second, or explosive, type of headache.

The third type of headache associated with sexual activity is the postural type and resembles that seen after the development of low cerebral spinal fluid, such as after a lumbar puncture. It is thought that it may be secondary to a dural leak during coitus/orgasm. This headache increases on standing. It is typically irregular in nature and not usually predictable. If it is regular, a trial of propranolol, between 40 and 240 mg a day, may be initiated. The beta-blocker may help by decreasing the surge of blood pressure at the time of orgasm. One difficulty with this treatment is that propranolol may decrease libido. Calcium channel blockers have also been tried.

Post-lumbar puncture headache

The post-lumbar puncture headache is a bilateral headache which develops any time up to 7 days after a lumbar puncture. The headache may be absent in the reclining patient and begin or worsen when the patient sits or stands, then decreasing in intensity or disappearing altogether when the patient again resumes a recumbent position. The apparent pathophysiology of the post-lumbar puncture is a leakage of cerebral spinal fluid (CSF) through the dural tear or puncture. When the volume of CSF is decreased (associated with decreased CSF pressure), the brain sags downward, affecting the pain-sensitive structures in the cranium, by traction, including the sagittal sinus and its tributary veins, as well as the large arteries at the base of the skull and the tentorium. Typically, the headache is self limiting, with a duration of less than 14 days. It may be prevented by having the patient remain lying on his stomach for 6 to 8 hours after lumbar puncture. If the headache occurs, fluids should be pushed. A blood patch, using the patient's blood, may be applied over the site of the initial lumbar puncture.

Postcarotid endarterectomy headache

Postcarotid endarterectomy headache may follow a thromboendarterectomy or other surgery of the extracranial carotid artery which has not dissected and is patent. It may begin within 2 days after surgery and is ipsilateral. It may last for days to months. The most common type of headache is mild, diffuse, and nonspecific in nature and begins within 5 days of surgery. There may also be ipsilateral "cluster-like headache" possibly secondary to surgical damage to the sympathetic nerve chain, but this is rare. The third type is severe, unilateral throbbing headache with associated increased arterial pressure, seizure, and focal neurological deficits. This is also rare and can foretell a cerebral hemorrhage.

Headaches associated with the eyes, ears, and sinuses

Headaches associated with ocular pathology are related to various difficulties. The first is acute open-angle glaucoma, which is associated with increased intraocular pressure. Glaucoma secondary to acute primary angle closure may have more serious consequences and should be ruled out.

Ocular inflammation may be secondary to non-granulomatous or granulomatous disorders. Granulomatous ocular inflammation may be slow or chronic in nature, with minimal pain. Sarcoidosis and tuberculosis are typical causes. This type is relatively rare.

The more common problem is the non-granulomatous inflammation. Pain may be minimal to severe and related to the inflammation or to a secondary increase in intraocular pressure. Complaints of earache, toothache, and sinus pain as well as tearing and blepharospasm are common. Of interest, diagnostically, is that light stimulation to the non-involved eye will cause pain in the affected eye. Scleritis and corneal abrasions may be associated with pain. Optic neuritis is frequently associated with pain on eye movement, secondary to the close attachments of the rectus muscles to the optic nerve sheath at the apex of the orbit.

Eye strain, or asthenopia, is noted to be a much less well-defined cause of headache than many may think. In one study, it was noted that among 50 patients with recent onset of presbyopia, only 6 had headache with near tasks, and 3 of these patients had improvement with correction.[330]

Pain in the ear may be associated with headache. Pain from the outer ear may be referred to the temporal or parietal regions or to the vertex. Its cause is typically visible. Pain from within the ear is more difficult to diagnose, and such otalgia may indicate the need for a more thorough evaluation including tomography and MRI. More common causes include mastoiditis and otitis media, which are relatively simple to diagnose.

Sinus disease may be associated with headache. Diagnostic criteria from the International Headache Society[12] include: purulent discharge in the nasal passage either spontaneously or by suction, pathological findings on one or more tests (X-ray, CAT scan, or MRI), transillumination, and the simultaneous onset of headache and sinusitis. In acute frontal sinusitis, the headache is located directly over the sinus and may radiate to the vertex or behind the eyes; in acute maxillary sinusitis, the headache is located over the antral area and may radiate to the upper teeth or the forehead; in acute ethmoiditis, the headache is located between and behind the eyes and may radiate to the temporal region; and in acute sphenoiditis, the headache is located in the occipital area, the vertex, the frontal region, or behind the eyes. The headache will disappear after treatment of the acute sinusitis. Commonly, testing will reveal an increase in white blood cells on CBC with a left shift. Treatment, aside from simple analgesics, should include a decongestant and an antibiotic.

Headache associated with acute and chronic substance usage

As discussed earlier, headache may be associated with a single use of substances. If secondary to toxic-metabolic substances, these headaches are typically generalized, persistent, throbbing, and associated with increased intensity with increased dosage of substances. These substances may include nitrates and nitrites, nitroglycerin, monosodium glutamate, carbon monoxide, alcohol, aspartame, phenylethylamine, tyramine, cocaine/crack, heavy metals, organophosphates, and nicotine. Headache from substance withdrawal may follow cessation of alcohol, birth control pills, or estrogens.

Headache may also be associated with chronic use of medications and other substances. The most common problems include the aforementioned analgesic rebound and vasoconstrictor rebound headaches from analgesics and the ergots and other forms of vasoconstrictor medications. When these medications are simply stopped, the patient will develop a rebound headache (typically more severe than the daily headaches they were experiencing) which may last 2 to 4 days.

One must not forget the other symptoms and medical problems which chronic medication (of the types noted immediately above) may induce. These may include ergotism or ergotamine toxicity, as well as nephropathy and cardiovascular, hematological, and gastrointestinal disorders. Prevention by clinicians is probably of greater importance than anything else. There are various methods used to detoxify patients, with the previously noted intravenous metaclopramide and DHE-45 protocol having the greatest effectiveness.

AH HA! *A major mistake made all too frequently is the belief that just getting rid of the offending medications will help the patient "enough". While it is true that stopping chronic analgesic or vasoconstrictive medication intake will help the typical patient by 40 to 60%, at least initially, if nothing more is done to help the patient's initial headache problem, for which they started the medications, it will continue, and the patients will re-start their medication intake with over-the-counter analgesics, or will visit another physician. The clinician should be prepared to treat their patients immediately with prophylactic medications, if appropriate, or physical therapy for tension-type headaches, psychotherapy for depression (with or without antidepressant medications), and possibly biofeedback-enhanced neuromuscular re-education and stress reduction.*

That being said, let's move on to the next chapter which deals with the interdisciplinary treatment of headache.

chapter twelve

Interdisciplinary treatment of headache

The majority of headache patients are seen most often in the office of their primary care physician or chiropractor, and their treatment typically goes very well. As a headache specialist, one sees the 20 to 25% of patients who do not do well initially, which is as it should be. The author, for instance, is not a specialist in hearts, lungs, livers, and so on, so patients with those types of medical problems (and a lot of others) are referred back to the their primary care physicians or to specialists.

The bottom line is that headache specialists in headache clinics see the tough patients, for the most part. Sure, some early post-traumatic headaches or out-of-control migraine or cluster patients are seen, as well as patients who skipped their primary care physicians because they were fearful of a brain tumor. But, mostly, the patients have "been there, done that" and are fed up with doctors, headache pain, and the system, whichever one they are enrolled in. This means that they may be angry, suspicious, and even downright hostile. And, in many cases, I cannot blame them.

And now they come into this center which specializes in the treatment of headache and pain. An end-of-the-road place. The last-chance gas station. They expect more of the same thing they received before — no help, just a money sink. So, the first thing that must be done is to change their perceptions of where they are, why they are there, and what can be done to help them.

"How," you may ask, "do we do that?" Well, the process begins when they first walk through the door into your office. In my practice, we try to get as much information regarding insurance, referral source, and so on over the phone when they first call. There is therefore a minimal amount of paper work to be done when they arrive. The office should be calm, so the patient does not feel uncomfortable. After signing in, the patient is met by "his" internal nurse case manager, an R.N. who has been specifically trained to work with headache and pain patients and who has the medical and psychological knowledge to help them feel comfortable. This nurse then takes a thorough history, utilizing a 15-page, copyrighted form developed over 16 years. This may take an hour, or even two.

Then the physician goes over the patient's past medical records, lab tests and scans, and the fresh history with the nurse that took it. The physician then meets with the patient and goes over the history form again, verifying some points and having the patient further expound upon specific information as needed.

The patient then is examined neurologically and musculoskeletally, with aspects of orthopedic and physical medicine examinations utilized as needed. Physical findings are pointed out to the patient in the examination room, where the beginning of the patient's education process has started. After the examination, the patient is seen again in the physician's office, with the internal nurse case manager. The results of the examination and the diagnoses are explained again, and the patient is allowed to ask any questions he may still have.

A treatment plan is decided on, with the patient's approval. Medications which are prescribed are explained in detail, particularly as to why the physician wants to use them and what side effects may be expected. Medication refills are not given. Each and every refill must be called in from the patient's pharmacy. It is then written on the patient's pharmacy record in their nursing chart. This enables the nurse and physician to know if the patient is taking his medication correctly and on a timely basis.

It is made clear to the patient that their initial contact person for any questions or problems they may encounter is the nurse who took the patient's history and, if the patient is a woman, who was present during the examination. The process takes 2 to 3 hours, on average.

During the last part of their evaluation, when the patient is meeting again with the physician and their nurse, the physician takes the time to explain in detail what is going on with the patient physiologically and gives the patient reprints of published articles which the patient can take home.

At the conclusion of the evaluation, the patient, although still possibly hesitant, is at least ready to return to the clinic to see what will happen. At least 70% of these patients have stated that they have never received such a thorough evaluation. They are allowed to talk to a medical person and get whatever they want to off of their chest. They like it, for the most part. We explain that we are not there to "cure" them, but rather to help them help themselves. The patient is empowered.

They feel listened to and, for the most part (if possible), physically vindicated by the findings on their examination which were explained to them. They have pertinent information to take home and share with their spouses and significant others. Many of the patients who are seen have already been tested so much that they think they should be glowing in the dark. They are relieved that such tests do not have to be repeated.

> **AH HA!** *Some headache specialty clinics perform a battery of tests on all new patients. Some clinics will perform an EEG, an MMPI, facial thermography, and carotid and temporal artery doppler blood flow studies. All this, even before the patient sees the physician! To put it nicely, it ain't necessary! As previously noted, a true headache specialist should know the diagnosis after the history and examination at least 98% of the time. Such tests in this situation are done purely for monetary gain. They simply should not be. If, after the history and examination, seizures are suspected, an EEG should be done. If the patient is depressed, an MMPI should be done after meeting with a psychologist who verifies that the testing should be done. Facial thermography is done to see the ipsilateral "cold spot" in cluster headache patients. If a headache specialist cannot diagnose cluster headache from the history, even without the neurological examination, he is not a headache specialist.*

The essence of the interdisciplinary treatment team (ITT) approach is that there is one medical "captain of the ship" who diagnoses, treats, and works with the clinical staff to enable timely, cost-effective diagnosis and treatment so that the patient gets better. To run an ITT, the clinician *must* know enough about each of the other specialties involved that he is able to help the various team members in their treatment approaches if and when needed.

The other members of the headache treatment team should include physical therapists, psychotherapists, biofeedback therapists, and, in the author's clinic, a chiropractor. Having an on-site interventional anesthesiologist is also quite helpful. Oh, yes, the term "on-site" is very important. To require patients to be treated in two or more facilities so that they have to drive around town with their headaches and their feelings of aggravation is certainly not optimal. The patients resent it. Communication between all treating clinicians is typically poor, which is also detrimental to good patient outcome. It is better by far to have all aspects of a patient's treatment under one roof. There is no substitute for the type of care given nor the speed at which important communication can take place in such a facility.

Weekly staff meetings involving all treating staff should be held. Questions about the patient's progress can then be discussed and changes in treatment ordered. Even more importantly, if there is a significant problem or medication reaction (significant or not), then the nurse or physical therapist or whomever can speak to the physician within minutes, sooner if there is an emergency. You never know what can come up. You just have to expect anything.

Case histories

The first is short and sweet. The superb chiropractor working with the author was seeing a female patient

> referred to him by the physical therapy department. He interrupted me during a consultation and asked me to see the patient, who he had been examining for the first time in almost a month, as she had had family problems. He was suspicious of another problem in her calf muscle, and he was absolutely correct. The patient had all the signs and symptoms of a deep venous thrombosis. Her personal family physician was called and advised of our concerns, and the patient was taken to his office. He hospitalized her, and heparin was started after further testing verified the diagnosis — all within 4 hours of the chiropractic physician seeing the patient and asking for my second opinion. That is satisfying.
>
> Another patient with a diagnosis of post-traumatic headache was seeing the neuropsychologist in my clinic for neuropsychological testing. The neuropsychologist noted the patient was having staring spells which had not been witnessed by anyone else, nor was there a corresponding history of them reported by the patient or his wife. The patient was seen a half hour later by the author, in the presence of the neuropsychologist, and we discussed the potential problems, specifically of the presence of partial complex seizures. Repeat neurological examination was negative. An EEG was ordered, and the patient was placed on carbamazepine. Within a week, his cognitive problems were somewhat resolved (but certainly not completely, as he had minor traumatic brain injury), and the "staring spells" stopped.

Earlier in this book I mentioned a patient who told his physical therapist of his suicidal ideation. Again, intervention took less than an hour. I could go on and on, but why? You get the point.

It is this author's bias that patients should receive the best care given by the most qualified practitioners. Therefore, we have registered physical therapists and physical therapy assistants in our clinic. The clinical psychologist and the neuropsychologist are both doctorate level. The biofeedback therapist has received certification. The nurses are experienced and act as the glue to keep everything going smoothly. Every clinician is in agreement with the clinic's treatment philosophies, including that of the ITT. The therapists are not told what to do, but they are allowed to use their experience and intelligence. The physician is there whenever needed. If a physical therapist speaks to me about getting a shoulder sonogram, I will approve it, as I trust her judgment.

We have also found that having chiropractic input into the ITT is extremely helpful. The fact that none of the other clinicians have pre-set notions or negative feelings about chiropractic treatment is extremely important, as otherwise the team as a whole could not function appropriately.

So, what do the other parts of the team do, aside from the obvious? The physical therapist is important in the treatment of headache secondary to soft tissue difficulties or a myofascial pain syndrome. Some physical therapists, utilizing company (insurance, HMO, or PPO) or other medical protocols, will immediately start a patient exercising and conditioning. Clinically, this is inappropriate. If a patient has a great deal of muscle spasm, forcing the muscle to work harder will reinforce the spasm and pain. The spasm must be released before significant work can be done by the musculature. Modalities may be needed initially to enable the spasm to break.

Frequently, trigger point injections with 1 cc of 1% lidocaine without epinephrine may be needed to help break a particularly stubborn trigger point. When this is done, it should be *immediately* followed by physical therapy. No more than four to six trigger points should be injected at a time, no more than weekly for 3 weeks for a particular set of trigger points.

As soon as possible, the patient should be taught stretching exercises, given pictures of them, and told to perform them at least 2 to 3 times per day. Once the spasm is under control, strengthening and conditioning should be performed, with the patient being responsible for performing their exercises out of the clinic facility.

Biofeedback-enhanced neuromuscular re-education and relaxation, as well as stress reduction, are also important modalities which serve again to teach the patient exercises and techniques that they can perform by themselves at home. There are four types of biofeedback: EMG, or muscular; thermal, or temperature; galvanic skin response (GSR); and EEG, which is not utilized for headache treatment.

The point of biofeedback is that feedback is given immediately to a patient on a computer screen. The feedback tells the patient what is going on. He can see how high his muscle tension, or spasm is, via a surface EMG lead attached to specific musculature and connected to a computer with special biofeedback software. Then, when he performs a specific muscle relaxation exercise, he can get immediate feedback from watching the screen as to how well he has done by seeing how much the muscle relaxed. The patient can thus learn specific exercises and see that they are being performed correctly thanks to the the visual feedback (or auditory feedback) received immediately.

Biofeedback to control temperature was first started for the purpose of teaching people to reduce their blood pressure by warming (vasodilating the vessels) in their hands. It was totally unexpected to discover that patients doing this could abort a migraine when they had the aura to the migraine. This was a totally coincidental finding, which led to the use of thermal biofeedback for migraine headache.

Biofeedback for generalized stress reduction or GSR biofeedback has also been used for years. Patients learn exercises which can decrease the amount of GSR response on their skin and promote relaxation. Visualizations may be helpful with this technique. In 1996, a presidential medical task sorce announced findings that biofeedback was a legitimate therapeutic modality.

Psychotherapy is a two-edged sword. It is extremely important to deal with a chronic headache patient's affective difficulties, such as depression and anxiety. This must be done in a fashion that is not disagreeable to the patient. At first, particularly if a patient has no concept of his depression (pretty common, that!), he may be against the idea, as it may seem to him that the physician is telling him that his headaches are all "in his head". You cannot force a patient to do any particular therapy (or anything else, for that matter), so you have to convince them through education as to why psychotherapy would be helpful. The figures in the tension-type headache chapters showing that affective difficulties are natural occurrences in the face of chronic headache may help.

It is rare to find headache that is mostly psychological, and these patients typically resist the thought of working in psychotherapy. In such cases, a very limited number of physical therapy treatments given when he begins psychotherapy may be helpful, as it indicates to the patient that you, the clinician, are dealing with his physical problems, which the patient will understand, while the psychotherapy is begun simply as a "secondary treatment".

As noted in the chapter on the psychology of headache, there may be a significant number of headache/pain-related psychological difficulties which need to be worked on. If you will not or cannot perform treatment dealing with a patient's affective difficulties, when needed, you will not be able to help the patient to a significant, long-term degree.

The chiropractic aspect of care is important for a number of reasons. First, many patients feel that is the only way to go. It is then up to the chiropractor who begins treatment with the patient to educate them on why other aspects of treatment are important and to help the patient to be inclined to accept other types of care. Second, while there are limits to chiropractic treatment, there are also limits to physical therapy. Both types of clinicians working together will better help a patient achieve a headache-free status. It is better than trying to argue about which is better with patients. You must have an expert physical therapist who is not afraid to utilize chiropractic manipulation when it is appropriate. Many physical therapists have a negative mindset towards chiropractic, so you want to work with one who is experienced enough to know better than that. Particularly when dealing with joints and the vertebrae, up from the sacroiliac joint, physical therapists should know when their ability to deal with problems on a soft-tissue basis has reached its limit. On the other hand, chiropractic treatment should be short term (as should all treatment). Patients tend to develop a dependency on a clinician who sees them three or more times a week for months on end.

Remember, the point of treatment is to diagnose the headache problem, treat it, and educate the patient enough to enable him to stop over-utilization of medical services and medications. In reality, the vast majority of patients prefer it that way, as it gives them the control they need over their headaches, if they continue, and over their mind and body.

The interventional anesthesiologist may be very helpful with chronic headache patients, some of whom are so tender, they claim, that the physical therapist cannot even touch them. In patients with cervical myofascial pain syndrome, a C_2 ganglion block will create significant pain relief and allow the physical therapist to begin treatment. This particular block is also a good way to determine, in those rare cases, if the patient is being honest with you. A good C_2 ganglion block will induce pain relief in the cervical region; if done correctly, it has to, as the site of relayed cervical nociception has been temporarily turned off. If a patient still complains of pain which has not changed at all, you may have another diagnosis. In the case of discogenic disease, epidural steroid injections may also help shorten treatment time and cost, when combined with physical therapy.

The nurses, as noted above, help keep everything together. They are the patients' contact person, as well as their advocate. It is part of their job to make certain that any tests or procedures ordered are carried out. They also, most frequently, have the time to talk with patients about new or ancillary problems which have just come to the forefront, when there is a week or more before they are scheduled to see the physician. The nurse should talk to the physician as soon as possible to discuss the new information and determine if a change of treatment should be ordered.

The physician should be up to date on all patient problems. He should be made aware of any substantive changes in a patient's physical or emotional healing. As the "captain" of the medical ship, the physician should know whenever any of the other treating clinicians run into something new or find that their treatment is going exceptionally well or not as well as would have been expected. In the latter case, the physician must find out why. Is there a problem with the treatment, the patient's acceptance of the treatment, or even the diagnosis?

> **AH HA!** *Years ago I realized this: as you treat them, so shall you diagnose them! After your initial diagnosis, something else may rear its ugly head — i.e., another diagnosis. If treatment is appropriate for the correct diagnosis, but the patient is not getting better, stop treatment and re-assess the patient. Start from scratch if you have to. Most frequently you will find that your initial diagnosis was correct, but something else is there, physiologically or emotionally, which you did not see or was not there to see when you initially evaluated the patient. Recognize the new problem/diagnosis and change your treatment plan to encompass it.*

Now, a few words about medications. They were discussed in nauseating detail in earlier chapters. You should now know how and when to use them. But, a few comments must be made for the benefit of chiropractic physicians. In reading the last few years of chiropractic literature, it is obvious, if not blatantly obvious, that many chiropractors do not believe in medication usage. In fact, prescription medications of almost any type are felt to be "poisons" to some chiropractors. To some members of the chiropractic profession, this point represents the major difference between the practices of medicine and chiropractic.

Any medication, prescription or otherwise, if used incorrectly, may indeed become a poison to the patient. Or to anyone. In working as part of an interdisciplinary treatment team, the chiropractor must accept that there are other ways, not chiropractic necessarily, that can help a patient. In fact, clinical experience, as well as literature, shows that the adjunctive use of medication will help in treatment, by decreasing both the time and cost of overall treatment. If a patient has a decrease or dysmodulation of the brain's serotonergic system, medication is indicated to help restore normal neurochemical homeostasis.

As with the other members of the interdisciplinary treatment team who must acknowledge and utilize the chiropractor's knowledge and expertise, the chiropractor must perform or behave in the same manner. The entire essence of the interdisciplinary treatment team is to utilize the best from all of the involved treating clinician's fields. Otherwise, why bother?

A cautionary tale

We, as clinicians are doing what we do to help patients get better — specifically, in terms of this book, ameliorate or stop their headaches. But is that always what should be done? Both the allopathic and chiropractic medicine answers are "of course!" Unfortunately, that may not always be true.

You may remember from our earlier discussion on the psychology of headache that patients may have various psychological reasons for enduring their headaches. The headaches, over time, have become the entire focus of their lives. And we "smart" headache specialists are just going to disregard this fact and make them better in spite of themselves? Not a good idea.

In the case of a patient we will refer to as JM, who had spent 2 years enduring terrible headache pain, he was initially seen and multiple iatrogenic medical problems were dealt with. Then his headache was appropriately treated, and the patient became headache free. Was he happy? Well, let's put it this way. He attempted suicide. Why? The headaches had been the reason JM did not have to mobilize himself to attempt to return to school, something he felt he could not do well, but something that was expected of him by his family.

So, we got rid of his headaches and he had nothing left to hide behind. He was afraid of being exposed as a "loser" who couldn't hack it in school.

Prior to that realization, he had his severe headaches to keep him from going to school. When they were gone, he felt he was expected to perform, but he did not think he could. So he overdosed on calcium channel blockers, something that would give him a cardiac-pulmonary arrest.

Something else came out of this, too. To ask the patient why he had not been seen in several weeks, this physician called him. The patient, on the phone, was hyperventilating and complaining of shortness of breath. He was able to tell me about talks he'd had with his *other* psychologist, who before that moment was unknown to this physician. 911 was called and the patient was hospitalized for 3 days, the first 2 in the intensive care unit.

This other psychologist was called. He felt that his patient was getting more depressed and had resented the fact that he was seeing a psychologist in my clinic. So, he had told the patient not to continue to follow up with us. And, he ignored the patient's increasing depression that began when his headaches were taken away. Nice guy. He didn't even bother to ask which hospital the patient had been taken to.

This case should not be considered an isolated incident, as variations of this story are not uncommon. We have learned several important points here. First, the patient was seeing another clinician who was not communicating with the ITT. Not a good idea. Second, when a patient does not show up for treatment, check it out. Third, and most important, there are very rare times when you may not want to be a hero and rip away a patient's pain. Especially if that pain is what is holding the patient together by preventing him from doing something he may not want to do or feel capable of doing.

That's correct. Sometimes, if you get a full understanding of a patient's pain and the psychological/emotional substrates underlying that pain, you may not want to rid the patient of the pain until you have shored up the walls that might collapse if you do decrease or eliminate that pain. That's why I insist that patients with a lot of real or implied medical and/or especially emotional baggage be treated only by the ITT, unless, of course, there are medical problems we do not deal with.

Because of a poorly motivated psychologist, this patient may have lost his life. And the guy did not even ask where the patient was hospitalized. After his release from the hospital, the patient was given a choice. Us or him. He chose us and is still pain free and back in school, doing well. Think about it, and above all else do no harm.

In the next chapter we will deal with nerve blocks and other forms of interventional anesthesiological treatment of specific headache and other head and facial pain syndromes.

chapter thirteen

Nerve blocks and other interventional procedures

The treatment and rehabilitation of headache are easy and conservative, right? Well, most commonly, that's right. The essential point, though, is that there are no "always" or "never" rules in practicing headache management.

A topic of great debate has been the utilization of the interventional anesthesiologist. These physicians have had specialized training in the use of nerve blocks in the diagnosis and treatment of nerve-related pain problems. However, there is a great deal more to it than that. To become a truly great maven of the diagnosis and treatment of headache and associated pain problems, one must know about all the tools that may be used and, most importantly, know when and why to use them.

Yes, some headache specialists do not like the idea of using needles on their patients. Few others understand that a tool is only as good as the role it plays in the final creation, the headache-free status of your patient. It is necessary to discuss the use of interventional procedures in the treatment of some types of headache and pain.

Tension-type headache

There are three or four occasions in the treatment of tension-type headache when one might think of using a needle. The first is in the treatment of the trigger points that were discussed in the chapter on the pathophysiology of tension-type headache. Trigger points are small areas of hypersensitivity in muscle which is involved in a myofascial pain syndrome. These painful areas are found in taut bands of skeletal muscle and are usually easy to palpate. When active, they are noted to refer pain in a myotomal distribution when they are palpated. Each time the trigger point is pressed, pain (or, rarely, paresthesias) is referred outwardly, to the same place. Trigger points have an "energy crisis" — a marked decrease of energy-producing chemicals — as well as decreased vascularity from compression and relative hypoxia. They produce, whether active or latent, muscle problems including decreased range of motion, weakness, and increased fatigability. So, to enable healing to occur and stop associated headache, they need to be irradicated, if at all possible. The first, conservative treatment is simple physical therapy. If this modality fails after three or four sessions, the next treatment should be trigger point injections.

These injections are commonly performed by all types of clinicians, who do so ably without a lot of training. A small-gauge needle is used to place anywhere from .5 to 1 cc of fluid, typically 1 or 2% lidocaine without epinephrine or bupivicaine with or without steroid. Sterile saline may be used, although patients may be more comfortable with the local anesthesia. Dry needling, which involves a larger gauge needle, typically is not a good idea in the head and neck with its higher degree of vascularity. Four to six trigger points may be injected at one sitting. Remember that too much anesthetic may induce side effects. The trigger points may require two or three injections, given at least a week apart. One of the important caveats is that immediately after the trigger point injections, the patients should receive ultrasound over the injected areas. This modality helps to further break down the trigger points and therefore aids in over all rehabilitation.

Some patients, particularly after cervical trauma such as an acceleration/deceleration injury, may be in too much pain for appropriate physical therapy to be used. They hurt too much, they will tell you, to be touched. If oral medications do not help this problem and it prevents the application of physical therapy, it may be necessary to perform a C_2 ganglion block. This should be done by a very experienced interventional anesthesiologist.

As the nociceptive input from much of the cervical and upper back and head regions passes through this ganglion to the spinal cord trigeminal nucleus, a well-performed block in this region, performed under fluoroscopy, will induce a numbness resulting in a pain-free patient who can then tolerate the physical therapy necessary to increase muscle relaxation and range of motion.

One aspect of this neural blockade is that it may help in the determination of patients who are consciously magnifying their complaints of pain/headache. These patients may have the block done by the best interventionalist in your area and still state that there is absolutely no reduction in pain. This means one of two things. Either the patient is malingering, or you missed something.

If the patient has been worked up and found not to have any other physiological difficulties, he may indeed be malingering, and treatment should be terminated. On the other hand, there may be a cervical spinal vertebral facet or joint problem which is referring pain in a sclerotomal distribution, which is different from myotomal or dermatomal distributions. In this situation, which will be discussed in great detail elsewhere, a facet joint injection, performed under fluoroscopy, should be performed. The bony/joint problem may be found on plain films or more sophisticated neuroimaging procedures such as a CAT scan. A patient should not be considered a malingerer until all possible sites of pain generation have been ruled out.

Another appropriate use for an interventional anesthesiological consult is when neuroimaging has revealed a small disc protrusion or herniation, with or without neural foraminal encroachment. Conservative rehabilitative treatment is very useful to help the patient avoid surgery, which may be necessary for a number of reasons. One excellent adjunctive treatment is a cervical epidural steroid injection, or a series of two to three injections over 2 to 3 weeks. This procedure may not produce immediate pain relief after the injected local anesthetic wears off. It may take days or weeks for the patient to begin to appreciate the effects of the injected steroid. The injections will also further enable physical therapy to be performed.

Remember that tension-type headache that does not respond as you would expect to conservative treatment, as outlined earlier, should be further evaluated to make certain that no other organic pathology has been missed, either a disc problem or a facet joint disruption.

Occipital neuralgia

Occipital neuralgia is a common cause of posterior cervical headache. Unfortunately, it is not a routine part of the differential diagnosis. Patients with occipital neuralgia typically complain of suboccipital pain that radiates up the back of the head or down the neck. It is possible to have retro-orbital radiation of pain secondary to the close proximity of the occipital nerve to the spinal nucleus of the trigeminal nerve. The pain may also be referred to the temporal regions. The cervical or headache pain may last for days or be only episodic.

Many patients experience occipital neuralgia as a burning, lancinating pain which lasts only a second or two at a time, but occurs frequently. Indomethacin is the treatment of choice for this problem. Occipital neuralgia may be confused with tension-type headache or pain secondary to trigger point radiation. Diagnostic nerve blocks of the greater occipital nerve at C_2 may be needed to help make the determination.

The greater occipital nerve of Arnold is the largest totally afferent nerve in the body. It forms from the posterior division of the II cervical nerve. It leaves the spinal column from between the arch of the atlas and axis, moves inferolaterally to the C_{2-3} facet (zygapophyseal) joint, ascends toward the occiput by moving around the inferior oblique capitis muscle, and then goes deep to the semispinalis capitis muscle. It pierces through the tendinous insertion of the trapezius muscle to between the trapezius and semispinalis muscle and then arrives at the subcutaneous tissue of the occipital region.

The lesser occipital nerve is derived from the anterior divisions of the II and III cranial nerves. It ascends more directly by following the posterior margin of the sternocleidomastoid muscle. It provides sensation to the scalp regions lateral to the region innervated by the greater occipital nerve.

The most common problem inducing occipital neuralgia is entrapment neuropathy. This can occur either near the origin of the nerve root as it exits the spine from direct nerve root compression by the inferior oblique capitis muscle or at the C_{2-3} facet joint. The second region for entrapment is in the sub-occipital region, where it might be compressed by muscle spasm.

Other discrete problems such as cervical spondylosis or a ruptured cervical disc may induce a secondary occipital neuralgia from reflexively spasmed muscles.

Nerve entrapment near the cervical spine should induce increased symptoms during extension or rotation of the head and neck, alone or with compression of the skull on the neck. Entrapment of the nerve as it moves through the tendinous insertion of the trapezius muscle on the skull is more likely to cause pain during neck flexion.

Cervical facet blocks, as well as occipital nerve blocks, are useful once the area of the entrapment has been delineated. Neurolytic blocks are frequently found to cause deafferentation neuralgia. Cryoneurolysis of the occipital nerve is more effective but may require a surgical exposure of the nerve.

Sphenopalatine neuralgia

Sphenopalatine neuralgia may frequently be confused with cluster headache based on some similarities between the two. It was first described in the early 1900s and is very painful, with the pain described as burning or aching and located in the peri-orbital and retro-orbital region, which may include the temple, maxilla, and upper gum. It typically has ipsilateral rhinorrhea, lacrimation, and injected conjunctiva, similar to cluster headache. Unlike cluster, though, sphenopalatine neuralgia is more common in woman than men and usually begins during the third to fifth decades of life.

Unlike the short-lived cluster headache (45 to 90 minutes), the headaches from sphenopalatine neuralgia may last hours to days. The burning and aching pain of sphenopalatine neuralgia differs from the pain of cluster headache, most frequently described as boring, stabbing, or shooting.

The sphenopalatine ganglion, which is found submucosally in the lateral wall of the nasopharynx, may be blocked by local anesthetic applied in the nasopharynx over the surface of the ganglion. Topical anesthetic (2% lidocaine) on cotton-tipped applicators may be used. In the past, cocaine was used for this purpose.

Neuroablative lesions of the sphenopalatine ganglion typically require injection into the pterygopalatine fossa of alcohol or phenol, but this procedure is not without the possibility of complications. Radiofrequency thermocoagulation of the sphenopalatine ganglion is as effective and poses fewer risks. Cryoneurolysis has also been used.

Trigeminal neuralgia

This clinical entity was discussed earlier in this book. The most common cause of trigeminal neuralgia is compression of the intracranial portion of the V cranial nerve. The offending vessels may include the superior cerebellar artery, the anterior and posterior cerebellar arteries, and also some veins.

Non-surgical treatment begun after conservative treatment has failed includes several interventional techniques. These include local anesthetic blockade of the gasserian ganglion as well as neuroablation with phenol or ethyl alcohol, which may induce significant side effects, including corneal anesthesia and anesthesia dolorosa, or a "painful numbness".

Safer for the patient is percutaneous retrogasserian glycerol rhizolysis (PRGR), during which glycerol is injected into the trigeminal cistern, inducing neurolysis of the gasserian ganglion and its central rootlets. Radiofrequency coagulation of the gasserian ganglion is also done, with fewer side effects. In both PRGR and radiofrequency lesioning, hypertension and tachycardia are frequent side effects.

One of the safest procedures is percutaneous balloon microcompression of the gasserian ganglion, which produces less sensory loss as well as lower incidence of anesthesia dolorosa.

These procedures are highly specialized and should be done by experienced interventional anesthesiologists. When appropriately incorporated into a patient's treatment, these procedures, and many more like them, can make diagnosis and overall treatment outcome much more favorable. In general, if needed, the use of interventional anesthesiology can make treatment move forward faster than treatment without the consultation. Time being money and all of that, it is therefore a good idea to have these procedures performed on your patients if needed, rather than just rely on the old standby medication and conservative rehabilitation alone.

In the next chapter, we will deal with something entirely different.

chapter fourteen

Cervicogenic headache: an introduction and manual medicine

We have already touched upon the importance of inclusion of interventional anesthesiological medicine as an adjunctive treatment for headache. In this chapter, we will discuss the concept of headache secondary to cervical spine problems — cervicogenic headache — as well as discuss the major proponents of this problem, the clinicians who treat headache with manual medicine. We will not be going into exhaustive detail here.

It is interesting to note that some headache specialists will deny the existence of cervicogenic headache. Many of these same clinicians will even deny the reality of muscle-related headache problems, including the existence of trigger points. Shortsighted, or overly focused on a narrow field of expertise? I couldn't tell you. The author does know, though, that to deny the existence of myofascial problems is, clinically, not helpful and exceptionally narrow minded.

The usefulness of manual medicine is also a major subject of debate. There are those who claim that conventional M.D. medicine is the end all and be all. There are those who accept M.D. medicine but add the usefulness of manual medicine — the osteopaths (D.O.). Then, at the other end of the spectrum, there are the Doctors of Chiropractic, many of whom attempt to differentiate themselves from everyone else by stating that, in effect, M.D. medicine, D.O. medicine, and the like are bad. The use of medications is felt to be the equivalent of poisoning patients. Manual medicine is the end all and be all. Unfortunately, these folk are as shortsighted as the others mentioned.

The key, the true end all and be all, is helping patients. If it takes a combination of conventional medicine, medication, rehabilitation, manual medicine and interventional medicine, what is the problem? As long as the patient gets better, who cares, as long as the treatment has been appropriate?

There does appear to be some things that manual medicine practitioners can do better than other clinicians. There are also things that conventional medicine can achieve that cannot be achieved by manual medicine alone. So, why not understand what each has to offer and utilize the best of each particular branch of medicine, when needed, to help patients? Seems to make sense, no?

Anyway, it is felt that the headache specialist should understand the other side of the coin and learn it well enough to utilize it to the patients' benefit. This is not to say that every patient will need manual medicine or interventional anesthesiology: they certainly do not! It is important to realize what other things are available and possibly appropriate to any individual patient.

The author is very fortunate in that he has superb physical therapists on his staff. These therapists, experts in what they do, are able to determine without prejudice when a patient may need a manual medicine consultation. They realize that there are some things at which they are not expert, and they call for the expert to do the work. The author is also lucky in having a superb Doctor of Chiropractic who works out of his clinic and sees patients when consulted. The patients receive the benefit of this more global view of their care and are quite pleased, as well as typically pain free, when treatment is over. So, lets look at some old things and some new things, with the idea that we can always learn something new, something which may help our patients.

Headache and the cranium

The International Headache Society[12] has specific diagnostic criteria for headache secondary to disorders of cranial bone. These criteria state that (1) there is clinical and/or laboratory evidence of a disorder in the cranium; (2) the headache is located in the affected cranial structure and radiates to its surroundings, and the pain may or may not be referred to more distant areas of the head; and (3) headache disappears within one month after successful treatment or spontaneous remission of the underlying disorder. The most frequent medical problems which can cause pain in the skull from lesions include multiple myeloma and osteomyelitis. The majority of skull lesions are asymptomatic.

Headache and the cervical spine

A number of cervical structures are equipped with nociceptors, including the apophyseal joints, the atlantooccipital (condylar) joints, the annulus fibrosis, the spinal ligaments, and vertebral periosteum, all parts of the vertebral column. The cervical musculature, the cervical nerve roots and nerves, and the vertebral arteries are also pain sensitive.

One outstanding headache specialist notes that three conditions should apply in order to implicate diseases or dysfunctions of the neck as a cause of headache:[342] (1) the cervical structures felt to be the source of the headache must be pain sensitive, (2) they must be located in an area where the "hard wiring" of the neural network permits referral of pain from that cervical focus to the head, and (3) the disease or dysfunctions involving those structures must be identifiable and verifiable.

It is also noted that there are limited ways pain may be referred to the head through the "hard wiring". As discussed earlier, these include: (1) stimulation of the C_2 sensory root and its extensions, the greater and lesser occipital nerves, which produces pain in the back of the head; (2) connections between the tentorial branches of the ophthalmic division of the Vth cranial nerve and the posterior fossa branches of C_2, which may allow referred pain from C_2-innervated structures to the front of the head; and (3) intermingling of nociceptive impulses from the upper cervical segments with those from cranial nerve VI, which may allow for referral of pain to the head. Additionally, although there is little evidence to believe in a C_1 sensory root,[343] if it does exist it may produce pain in the vertex or frontal aspects of the head.

As the spinal tract of the trigeminal nerve ends in the spinal cord between C_2 and C_4, it is unlikely that referral of pain from lower cervical regions would be able to refer pain to the head. This could be done via the first three or four cervical segments.

The International Headache Society diagnostic criteria for headaches associated with disorders of the cervical spine[12] include the presence of pain localized to neck and occipital regions, which may project to the forehead, orbital region, temples, vertex, or ears or pain precipitated or aggravated by special neck movements or sustained neck posture. At least one of the following occurs: resistance to or limitation of passive neck movements; changes in neck muscle contour, texture, tone, or response to active and passive stretching and contraction; and abnormal tenderness of neck muscles. Additionally, radiologic examination will reveal at least one of the following: movement abnormalities in flexion/extension, abnormal posture, and fractures, congenital abnormalities, bone tumors, rheumatoid arthritis, or other distinct pathology (not including spondylosis or osteochondrosis).

Among cervical etiologies of headache one may include developmental anomalies of the craniovertebral junction and upper cervical spine, including Arnold-Chiari malformation, with or without hydrocephalus. The headaches from craniovertebral anomalies appear to exhibit posterior location, triggering by flexing of the neck or by coughing and straining.[344] There may also be neurological signs and symptoms.

Trauma to the head or particularly forceful sneezing may induce rotatory subluxation of the atlas and, via irritation of synovial joints, persistent occipital headache. Rheumatoid arthritis of the upper cervical spine may cause inflammation of the synovial atlantooccipital and atlantoaxial joints, as well as stretching of the nerve roots and upper cervical ligaments secondary to atlantoaxial subluxation from attenuation of the transverse ligament of the odontoid. The occipital headache may be increased or set off by cervical movements or straining. When examining these patients, flexing or hyperflexing the neck may cause death secondary to compression of the medulla by the odontoid which is no longer bound to the atlas by the transverse ligament.

Cervical trauma via acceleration/deceleration injuries has been discussed earlier. Other aspects of it, however, include the possible compression of the C_1 or C_2 sensory roots between the occiput and the atlas, as well as the atlas and the axis.[345] Others attribute the emergence of post-traumatic migraine to axonal shearing, but not necessarily as part of the postconcussive syndrome.[346]

Cervicogenic headache

The concept of cervicogenic headache is also mired in debate with both total denial or full acceptance. Some proponents of the entity call it cervicogenic headache,[347] while others refer to it as vertebrogenic headache.[348] The former authors are led by Sjaastad and his group. They note that the headache profile for cervicogenic headache is that of unilateral headache pain which starts in the neck and is referred or spread to the oculo-fronto-temporo regions, which may be the site of maximal pain. The headache is nonthrobbing and moderate in severity. It may be episodic or continuous and may be provoked by neck movements or poor posture, or by pressure over the posterior neck or occiput. There may be nonradicular neck, shoulder, and arm pain. Sjaastad et al.[349] also note a female predominance with a history of head or neck trauma and transient relief from anesthetic blockade of the C_2 nerve root or the occipital nerve. Finally, they note nausea, vomiting, phono- and photophobia, blurred vision ipsilaterally, and problems swallowing.

Sjaastad and his group[349] also indicate that cervicogenic headache is a reaction pattern, not a disease entity. It may originate in any cervical bony structure or soft tissue. They feel that cervicogenic headache may be very common and possibly frequently thought to be migraine without aura.

The International Headache Society[12] has described cervicogenic headache as being pain felt primarily in the neck and occiput which may radiate anteriorly. It may be precipitated by certain neck movements or by sustained neck postures. There must be physical evidence of cervical disease or dysfunction such as resistance to or limitation of passive neck movements, palpable changes in the neck musculature, or abnormal tenderness in neck muscle. Radiological changes must be present in the neck such as abnormal posture, abnormalities in flexion/extension movements, or evidence of disease such as fracture, tumor, congenital anomaly, or rheumatoid arthritis, *not* including spondylosis or osteochondrosis (which are too common to have significant diagnostic significance).

Case study

TP, a 37-year-old, righthanded, white male was injured in a logging accident: his head struck a log and his neck hyperextended. There was a 30-minute loss of consciousness. He was injured 1.5 years before being seen. His chief complaint was severe and constant headache in the occipital region with episodic spread to the bitemporal regions. He had been treated by physical therapy and with medications, essentially all analgesics, before he was seen.

Examination revealed significant cervical muscle spasm and a markedly reduced cervical range of motion in all realms. Trapezius, deltoid, and paraspinus muscle spasms were found, as well as trigger points in these muscles and tenderness, increased tone, and trigger points in the pericranial, massetter, and sternocleidomastoid muscles. There were no neurological abnormalities found.

The patient was first carefully detoxified from his daily narcotics and simple analgesics. Then he was started in an interdisciplinary treatment program. Within a week it was noticed that his abilities to concentrate were poor, as was his memory. After 2 weeks of physical therapy, the patient had a markedly improved cervical range of motion, but he stated that his pain was no better. A C_2 ganglion block was performed under fluoroscopy and the patient stated he had minimal relief.

A repeat cervical MRI and plain films were done. There was nothing of note on these tests. The patient was then sent for a series of diagnostic cervical blocks. The patient reported cessation of his pain when the atlanto-axial (A-A) facet joint was injected with local anesthetic. Two more specific A-A facet blocks were performed with better than 70% relief each time (on a visual analogue scale). The patient would then drive home on a weekend (an 8-hour drive) or begin working on his house and complain of an immediate exacerbation of his pain.

When he found that the pain would be decreased by the A-A facet blocks, his depression also diminished. At that point, a neuropsychological evaluation was done, which demonstrated a mild traumatic brain injury. The patient did not want treatment for this problem. Because of continued exacerbations of his pain after he would perform functions which induced abnormal neck postures for extended periods of time, the atlano-axial joint was injected with phenol to induce neurolysis. When told it would take 3 to 4 weeks for maximal benefit, the patient became angry and left treatment, requesting more narcotics. The pain did diminish, according to the patient, as would be expected.

Secondary to the patient's mild traumatic brain injury, he was able to regain full cervical range of motion but still persisted in claiming a severe pain level, even after the phenol injection had time to perform neurolysis. The patient was noted to have pain in the appropriate sclerotomal distribution of the A-A joint. Interventional treatment was of obvious help in the determination of the specific facet joint problem, as well as its treatment. The major confounding variable was the patient's mild traumatic brain injury, which he did not want treated via instruction in compensatory strategies.

Manual medicine

Manual medicine is much better accepted in European countries than it is in the United States. The reasons for this are undoubtedly many, including the length of time it has been practiced there. Some of the techniques or procedures may be performed by the physical therapist, but all may be performed by the physician.[350] These techniques include high-velocity, low-amplitude thrusting procedures most commonly thought of as being characteristic of the manual medicine practitioner and known as "manipulation". These procedures are used to deal with an articulation and its related periarticular structures. They affect the joint mechanics as well as associated paravertebral musculature.

Articulatory procedures, or mobilization without impulse, use oscillatory repetitive motions in the direction of loss of motion, with gradual increases in the amount of force used. These procedures seem to influence the mechanical action of the articulation and its articular tissues. It also appears to influence the behavior of multiple types of mechanoreceptors associated with the articulation involved. Soft-tissue procedures, muscle energy techniques, myofascial release and function, and release by position techniques, along with articulatory procedures, are also performed by physical therapists.

The craniosacral procedures function via the inherently small amount of mobility between the skull and the spinal column. It is performed by applying force to the musculoskeletal system, especially to the skull and sacrum, to enhance physiological mobility and restore appropriate amplitude to the "cranial rhythmic pulse".

There are three essential models of manual treatment.[339] The first is known as the biomechanical model. It is a functional anatomical model and starts with the feet and moves to the head. The manual medicine approach restores the biomechanical relationship of each bone, joint, and muscle group in an effort to regain symmetrical mobility.

The neurological model indicates that the musculoskeletal system is an expression of CNS activity, as well as the point of afferent stimulation transmitted to the CNS for processing. The reflex model includes the effect of afferent mechanoreceptor musculoskeletal system activity which manifests itself in different ways. One is in the form of altered muscle activity such as early, tonic, or chronic skeletal muscle spasm. There is also output via the visceral structures which are affected by the autonomic nervous system.

Most important for our discussion of headache is the reflex control of the vasculature via the sympathetic nervous system. It is felt that manual restoration of more normal afferent mechanoreceptor activity has a primary influence on vasomotor tone via a somatovisceral reflex arc.

The third, or circulatory model, is thought to be effective in vascular headache. It is felt that maximizing biomechanical function of the cervical and upper thoracic spine will normalize neurological control of cerebral vasculature via the superior cervical ganglion, which controls the vasomotor tone for the head. The preganglionic fibers to the superior cervical ganglion come from the upper four thoracic segments and ascend in the cervical sympathetic trunk. Muscle spasm may also compress the venous and lymphatic vessels, and the return of normal venous circulation is also thought to be influenced by the cervical musculature.

The essential role of manual medicine is to restore maximum, pain-free movement of the musculoskeletal system, which has been returned to postural balance.[351] Manual medicine is a good adjunctive therapy to be used in combination with other medical treatment.[352] It has been noted to be clinically useful for headaches of many types.[353]

Research appears to indicate that manual medicine is most useful with tension-type headache and reputedly has a major role in the treatment of vascular headache. Specifically, myofascial release and craniosacral techniques early in the onset of migraine headache may abort the headache.[354,355] The postulated mechanism of action is the return of normal vasomotor tone.

Myofascial release, strain and counter-strain, muscle energy techniques, and soft-tissue mobilization have been identified as being useful in the treatment of the acute tension-type headache, as well as in maintenance. Manipulation and mobilization may also be used.[356] Maintenance treatment should also include an individualized exercise program. On an acute basis, the use of non-steroidal antiinflammatory medications is useful during treatment for a chronic postural or myofascial problem.

The usefulness of manual medicine has been only briefly touched on here, from the perspective of the chiropractic and, mostly, osteopathic schools. There are very interesting aspects of manual medicine from both schools of thought which are potentially as well as realistically useful in the treatment of headache. This introduction to manual medicine was presented to expose the reader to the full scope of the available treatment for headache. The full scope of treatment options should be recognized and understood by the headache specialist. That is the most sincere method to express caring for the headache patient.

Afterword

Well, that's about it. Almost all I know about headache, but, like my old Sensei used to say, I always hold back some tricks. As you read further and, through your practice, become a headache specialist (should you choose to), you will develop your own special "tricks" of the trade. Results of the important information I hope you have gleaned from this book should include:

1. You understand the pathophysiology of the various types of primary headache disorders.
2. You understand the medication and non-medication treatment of the primary headache disorders.
3. You understand that there is more to the treatment of headache than giving analgesic medications.
4. You have learned that there are some things not taught in medical school that may help your patients, i.e., manual medicine.
5. You have learned of the appropriateness of interventional anesthesiological procedures in the diagnosis and treatment of headache.

Headache treatment can be fun. It is one of the few areas of medicine where a major difference can be objectively made in a patient's life. You treat patients with the idea of helping them stop their headaches. When that happens, it is very rewarding. If you have learned the basics, such results should happen much more frequently than you would expect.

If you choose to specialize in the diagnosis and treatment of headache, it can be a good change to a good subspecialty. You must, however, begin to read the headache literature and never stop. The journals *Headache* and *Cephalalgia* are good places to start. As you will notice in the reference section, there are a lot of good research articles in non-headache-specific journals, as well. You should join the American Association for the Study of Headache and the American Academy of Pain Management, an interdisciplinary pain society.

You should also realize that the typical headache patient is outspoken. As a group, they are a force to be reckoned with. They are verbal, assertive, and have read a lot about their headache problems. You should be thankful for this, as it will help you to help them by being able to explain what is going on and why.

A very small percentage of patients afflicted with headache and other types of pain are in it for the drugs. It is a societal norm to expect pain medications for a pain problem. On the other hand, you have now learned how to treat headache without the use of analgesics.

You will need to make your stand when a managed care company tells you that it is less expensive and therefore better to treat headache patients with analgesics. Like a former United States first lady said, just say "no" and mean it. To do otherwise will entail giving your headache patients inappropriate care. Solutions to this problem, along with the correct way(s) to treat headache, are in this book. Show it to your patients. Remember it is your license, not theirs, that will get hit if appropriate treatment is not given. And headache patients are a verbal lot, with lots of local and regional and national groups.

Teach your associates the best ways to deal with headache. Most physicians who treat with analgesics do so because they do not know any other way, and they want to make their patients feel better. So help them. Teach them.

I've had the honor and distinct pleasure of lecturing on headache to physicians all over the country during the past 18 years. They are generally a good-natured lot, with a willingness to learn new things. I still find more things for me to learn, too. That is one of the many things that make it so much fun. There is no end to what you can learn about this subspecialty.

I am fascinated by the history of medicine, particularly the original articles written about headache, which is why I had to include them in this book. It is wonderful to see where we came from and compare it to where we are today in the diagnosis and especially the treatment of headache. I would be grateful for any tidbits of clinical knowledge or lore about headache not included in this book. Also, any other thoughts can be shared by sending them to the publisher.

Headache is a big problem — one of the most common problems to enter the offices of all types of practitioners. So, let's get useful information to the right places and allow it to be utilized. It will certainly help in your headache patients' care. In conclusion, thanks for spending the time with me. Until next time, be good to yourselves and your patients. So long for now.

References

1. Kandel, E.R. and Schwartz, J.H., *Principles of Neural Science*. Elsevier, New York, 1985, pp. 563–569.
2. Gilman, S. and Newman, S.W., *Manter and Gatz's Clinical Neuroanatomy and Neurophysiology*, 8th ed. F.A. Davis, Philadelphia, 1992, p. 140.
3. McHenry, L.C., *Garrison's History of Neurology*. Charles C Thomas, Springfield, IL, 1969.
4. Bille, B., Migraine in school children. *Acta Paediatr. Scand.*, 51(Suppl. 136):14–15, 1962.
5. Sacks O., *Migraine: Understanding a Common Disorder*. University of California Press, Berkeley, 1985.
6. Critchley, M., Migraine: from Cappadocia to Queen Square, in *Background to Migraine*, Vol. 1, Smith, R., Ed., Heinemann, London, 1967.
7. Liveing, E., *On Megrim, Sick Headache, and Some Allied Disorders: A Contribution to the Pathology of Nerve-Storms*. Churchill, London, 1873.
8. Dalassio, D.J., *Wolff's Headache, and Other Facial Pain*, 5th ed. Oxford University Press, New York, 1987.
9. Ziegler, D.K., Headache: a public health problem. *Neurol. Clin.*, 8:781–791, 1990.
10. Linet, M.S., Stewart, W.F., Celentano, D.D., Ziegler, D., and Sprecher, M., An epidemiologic study of headache among adolescents and young adults. *JAMA*, 261:2211–2216, 1989.
11. Mathew, N.T., Teuveni, U., and Perez, F., Transformed or evolutive migraine. *Headache*, 27:102–106, 1987.
12. Headache Classification Committee of the International Headache Society: Classification and diagnostic criteria for headache disorders, cranial neuralgia, and facial pain. *Cephalalgia*, 8(Suppl. 7):1–96, 1988
13. Ziegler, D.K. and Hassanein, R.S., Specific headache phenomena: their frequency and coincidence. *Headache*, 30:152–156, 1990.
14. Whitty, C.W.M., Migraine without headache. *Lancet*, ii:283–285, 1967.
15. Barrie, M.A., Fox, W.R., Weatherall, M., and Wilkinson, I.P., Analysis of symptoms of patients with headaches and their response to treatment with ergot derivatives. *Q. J. Med.*, 146:319–336, 1968.
16. Glista, G.G., Mellinger, J.F., and Rooke, E.D., Familial hemiplegic migraine. *Mayo Clin. Proc.*, 50:307–311, 1975.

17. Hanson, S.L., Borelli-Miller, L., Strange, P., Nielsen, B.M., and Olesen, J., Ophthalmoplegic migraine: diagnostic criteria, incidence of hospitalization, and possible etiology. *Acta Neurol. Scand.*, 81:54–60, 1990.
18. Fisher, C.M., Late-life migraine accompaniments as a cause of unexplained transient ischemic attacks. *Can. J. Neurol. Sci.*, 7:9–17, 1980.
19. Fisher, C.M., Late-life migraine accompaniments: further experience. *Stroke*, 17:1033–1042, 1986.
20. Rosenbaum, H.E., Familial hemiplegic migraine. *Neurology*, 10:164–170, 1960.
21. Kunkel, R.S., Migraine aura without headache. *Pain Manage.*, 3:176–182, 1990.
22. Emery, E.S., Acute confusional state in children with migraine. *Pediatrics*, 60:110–114, 1977.
23. Gascom, G. and Barlow, C., Juvenile migraine presenting as an acute confusional state. *Pediatrics*, 45:628–635, 1970.
24. Blau, J.N., Adult migraine: the patient observed, in *Migraine: Clinical and Research Aspects*, Blau, J.N. (Ed.) Johns Hopkins University Press, Baltimore, 1987.
25. Collaborative Group for the Study of Stroke in Young Women: Oral contraceptives and stroke in young women. *JAMA*, 231:718–722, 1975.
26. Moskowitz, M.A., The trigeminovascular system, in *The Headaches*, Olesen, J., Tfelt-Hansen, P., and Welch, K.M.A. (Eds.) Raven Press, New York, 1993, pp. 97–104.
27. Skinhoj, E. and Paulson, O.B., Regional blood flow in internal carotid distribution during migraine attack. *Br. Med. J.*, 3:569–570, 1969.
28. Hockaday, J.M. and Debney, L., The EEG in migraine, in *Basic Mechanisms of Headache*, Olesen, T. and Edvinsson, L. (Eds.) Elsevier, Amsterdam, 1988, pp. 365–376.
29. Jay, G.W., Epilepsy, migraine and EEG abnormalities in children: a review and hypothesis. *Headache*, 22:110–114, 1982.
30. Sicuteri, F., Testi, A., and Anselmi, B., Biomedical investigations in headache: increase in hydroxyindoleacetic acid excretion during migraine attacks. *Int. Arch. Allerg.*, 19:55–58, 1961.
31. Curran, D.A., Hinterberger, H., and Lance, J.W., Total plasma serotonin, 5-hydroxyindoleacetic acid and p-hydroxy-m-metholymandelic acid excretion in normal and migrainous subjects. *Brain*, 88:997–1010, 1965.
32. Raskin, N.H. and Knittle, S.C., Ice cream headache and orthostatic symptoms in patients with migraine headache. *Headache*, 16:222–225, 1976.
33. Raskin, N.H. and Schwartz, R.K., Ice-pick-like pain. *Neurology*, 30:203–205, 1980
34. Raskin, N.H., Hosobuchi, Y., and Lamb, S., Headache may arise from perturbation of brain. *Headache*, 27(8):416–420, 1987.
35. Weiller, C. et al., Brain stem activation in spontaneous human migraine attacks. *Nature Medicine*, 1(7):658–660, 1995.
36. Traurig, H.H. and Maley, G.E., The brain stem reticular core and monoamine system, in *Neuroscience in Medicine*, Conn, P.M. (Ed.) J.B. Lippincott, Philadelphia, 1995, pp. 227–235.
37. Goadsby, P.J., Uddman, R., and Edvinsson, L., Cerebral vasodilatation in the cat involves nitric oxide from parasympathetic nerves. *Brain Res.*, 707:110–118, 1996.

38. Goadsby, P.J., Zagami, A.S., and Lambert, G.A., Neural processing of craniovascular pain: a synthesis of the central structures involved in migraine. *Headache,* 31(6):365–371, 1991.
39. Ullmer, C. et al., Expression of serotonin receptor mRNAs in blood vessels. *FEBS Lett.,* 370(3):215–221, 1995.
40. Olesen, J., Thomsen, L.L., and Iversen, H., Nitric oxide is a key molecule in migraine and other vascular headaches. *Trends Pharmacol. Sci.,* 15:149–153, 1994.
41. Hoskin, K.L., Kaube, H., and Goadsby, P.J., Central activation of the trigeminovascular pathway in the cat is inhibited by dihydroergotamine: a c-Fos and electrophysiological study. *Brain,* 119:249–256, 1996.
42. Goadsby, P.J. and Olesen, J., Diagnosis and management of migraine, *Br. Med. J.,* 312:1279–1283, 1996.
43. Gebhart, G.F., Visceral pain mechanisms: relevance to migraine, in *Experimental Headache Models,* Olesen, J. and Moskowitz, M.A. (Eds.) J.B. Lippincott, Philadelphia , 1995, pp. 39–47.
44. Traurig, H.H. and Maley, B.E., The trigeminal system, in *Neuroscience in Medicine,* Conn, P.M. (Ed.) J.B. Lippincott, Philadelphia, 1995, pp. 239–248.
45. Hoyer, D., et al., Seventh International Union of Pharmacology classification of receptors for 5-hydroxytryptamine. *Pharmacol. Rev.,* 46:157–203, 1994.
46. Goadsby, P.J. and Edvinsson, L., Peripheral and central trigeminovascular activation in cat is blocked by the serotonin (5HT)-1D receptor agonist 311C90. *Headache,* 34:394–399, 1994.
47. Shepeard, S.L. et al., Comparison of the effects of sumatriptan and the NK1 antagonist CP-99,994 on plasma extravasation in dura mater and c-Fos mRNA expression in trigeminal nucleus caudalis of rats. *Neuropharmacology,* 34:255–261, 1995.
48. Romberg, M.H., *A Manual of Nervous Diseases of Man.* Syndenham Society, London, 1840 (translated by E.H. Sieveking).
49. Ekbom, K.A., Ergotamine tartrate orally by Horton's "histaminic cephalgia" (also called Harris' "ciliary neuralgia"). *Acta Psychiatr. Scand.,* 46(suppl.):106–113, 1947.
50. Kunkle, E.C., Pheiffer, J.B., Jr., Wilhoit, W.M., and Hamrick, L.W., Jr., Recurrent brief headache in "cluster" pattern. *Trans. Am. Neurol. Assoc.,* 77:240–243, 1952.
51. Kudrow, L., *Cluster Headache: Mechanisms and Management.* Oxford University Press, London, 1980, pp. 10–150.
52. Lovshin, L.L., Clinical caprices of histaminic cephalgia. *Headache,* 1:3–6, 1961.
53. Ekbom, K.A., A clinical comparison of cluster headache and migraine. *Acta Neurol. Scand.,* 46(Suppl. 41):1–48, 1970.
54. Kudrow, L., The cyclic relationship of natural illumination to cluster period frequency (abstract). *Cephalalgia,* 7(Suppl. 6):76–77, 1987.
55. Kudrow, L., Plasma testosterone levels in cluster headache: preliminary results. *Headache,* 16:28–31, 1976.
56. Klimek, A., Plasma testosterone levels in patients with cluster headache. *Headache,* 22:162–164, 1982.
57. Bussone, G., Frediani, F., Leone, M., Grazzi, L., Lamperti, E., and Boiardi, A., TRH test in cluster headache. *Headache,* 7:43–54, 1988.

58. Facchinetti, F., Nappi, G., Cicoli, C. et al., Reduced testosterone levels in cluster headache: a stress–related phenomenon. *Cephalalgia,* 6:29–34, 1986.
59. Polleri, A., Nappi, G., Murialdo, G., Bono, G., Martignoni, E., and Savoldi, G., Changes in the 24-hour prolactin pattern in cluster headache. *Cephalalgia,* 2:1–7, 1982.
60. Chazot, G., Claustrat, B., Grun, J., Jordan, D., Sassolas, G., and Schott, B., A chronobiological study of melatonin, cortisol, growth hormone and prolactin secretion in cluster headache. *Cephalalgia,* 4:213–220, 1984.
61. Waldenlind, E., Gustafsson, S.A., Ekbom, K., and Wetterbert, L., Circadian secretion of cortisol and melatonin in cluster headache during active cluster periods and remission. *J. Neurol. Neurosurg. Psychiatry,* 50:207–213, 1987.
62. Ferrari, E., Martignoni, E., Vailati, A., Nappi, G., Savoldi, G., and Mandelli, B., Chronobiological aspects of cluster headache: effect of lithium therapy, in *Headache,* Savoldi, F. and Nappi, G. (Eds.) Palladio Editore, Pavia, 1979, pp. 152–160.
63. Nappi, G., Facchinetti, G., Bono, G. et al., Lack of B–endorphin and B–lipotropin circadian rhythmicity in episodic cluster headache: a model for chronopathology, in *Updating in Headache,* Pfaffenrath, V., Lundberg, P.O., and Sjaastad, O. (Eds.) Springer–Verlag, Berlin, 1985.
64. Fanciullacci, M., Pietrini, U., Gatto, G., Boccuni, M., and Sicuteri, F., Latent dysautonomic pupillary lateralization in cluster headache. A pupillometric study. *Cephalalgia,* 2:135–144, 1982.
65. Kudrow, L., McGinty, D.S., Phillips, E.R., and Stevenson, M., Sleep apnea in cluster headache. *Cephalalgia,* 4:33–38, 1984.
66. Kudrow, L. and Kudrow, D.B., Association of sustained oxyhemoglobin desaturation and onset of cluster headache attacks. *Headache,* 30:474–480, 1990.
67. Sakai, F. and Meyer, J.S., Regional cerebral hemodynamics during migraine and cluster headaches measured by the 133Xe inhalation method. *Headache,* 18:122–132, 1978.
68. Lance, J.W. and Anthony, M., Thermographic studies in vascular headache. *Med. J. Aust.,* 1:240–243, 1971.
69. Drummond, P.D. and Anthony, M., Extracranial vascular responses to sublingual nitroglycerin and oxygen inhalation in cluster headache patients. *Headache,* 25:70–74, 1985.
70. Norris, J.W., Hachinski, V.C., and Cooper, P.W., Cerebral blood flow changes in cluster headache. *Acta Neurol. Scand.,* 54:371–374, 1976.
71. Ekbom, K.A. and Grietz, T., Carotid angiography in cluster headache. *Acta Radiol. (Diagn.),* 10:177–186, 1970.
72. Anthony, M. and Lance, J.W., Histamine and serotonin in cluster headache. *Arch. Neurol.,* 25:225–231, 1971.
73. Appenzeller, O., Becker, W., and Ragas, A., Cluster headache. Ultrastructural aspects. *Neurology,* 28:371, 1978
74. Appenzeller, O., Becker, W.J., and Tagaz, A., Cluster headache. Ultrastructural aspects and pathogenetic mechanisms. *Arch. Neurol.,* 38:302–306, 1981.
75. Liberski, P.P. and Prusinski, A., Further observations on the mast cells over the painful region in cluster headache patients. *Headache,* 22:115–117, 1982.
76. Liberski, P.P. and Mirtecka, B., Mast cells in cluster headache. Ultrastructure, release pattern, and possible pathogenetic significance. *Cephalalgia,* 4:101–106, 1984.

77. Cuypers, J., Westphal, K., and Bunge, S.T., Mast cells in cluster headache. *Acta Neurol. Scand.*, 61:327–329, 1980.
78. Aebelholt–Krabbe, A. and Rank, F., Histological examinations of the superficial temporal artery in patients suffering from cluster headache. *Cephalalgia*, 5(Suppl. 3): 282–283, 1985.
79. Sicuteri, F., Fanciullacci, M., Geppetti, P., Renzi, D., Caleri, D., and Spillantini, M.G., Substance P mechanism in cluster headache evaluation in plasma and cerebrospinal fluid. *Cephalalgia*, 5:143–149, 1985.
80. Sicuteri, F., Geppetti, P., Marabini, S., and Lembeck, F., Pain relief by somatostatin in attacks of cluster headache. *Pain*, 18:359–365, 1984.
81. Moskowitz, M.A., The neurobiology of vascular head pain. *Ann. Neurol.*, 16:157–168, 1984.
82. Stowell, A., Physiologic mechanisms and treatment of histaminic or petrosal neuralgia. *Headache*, 9:187–194, 1970.
83. Dimitriadou, V., Henry, P., Brochet, B., Mathiau, P., and Aubineau, P., Cluster headache: ultrastructural evidence for mast cell degranulation and interaction with nerve fibres in the human temporal artery. *Cephalalgia*, 10:221–228, 1990.
84. Jay, G.W., Pathophysiology of tension–type headache, in *Headache: Diagnosis and Treatment*, Tollison, C.D. and Kunkle, R.S. (Eds.) Williams & Wilkins, Baltimore, 1993, p. 129.
85. Speed, W.G., Muscle contraction headaches, in *Headache Disorders*, Saper, J.R. (Ed.) John Wright, Boston, 1983, p. 115.
86. Diamond, S. and Dalessio, D.J., *The Practicing Physician's Approach to Headache*, 3rd ed. Williams & Wilkins, Baltimore, 1980.
87. Dorpat, T.L. and Holmes, T.H., Mechanisms of skeletal muscle pain and fatigue. *Arch. Neurol. Psychiatry*, 74:628, 1955.
88. Perl, S., Markle, P., and Katz, L.N., Factors involved in the production of skeletal muscle pain. *Arch. Intern. Med.*, 53:814, 1934.
89. Hong, S., Kniffki, K., and Schmidt, R., *Pain Abstracts*, Second World Congress on Pain, 1978, p. 58.
90. Rodbard, S., Pain associated with muscle contraction. *Headache*, 10:105, 1970.
91. Martin, P.R. and Mathews, A.M., Tension headaches: psychophysiological investigation and treatment. *J. Psychosom. Res.*, 22:389, 1978.
92. Sakuta, M., Significance of flexed posture and neck instability as a cause of chronic muscle contraction headache. *Rinsho Shinkeigato*, 30:254, 1990.
93. Riley, T.L., Muscle–contraction headache. *Neurol. Clin.*, 1:489, 1983
94. Philips, C., Tension headache: theoretical problems. *Behav. Res. Ther.*, 16:249, 1978.
95. Philips, C. and Hunter, M.S., A psychophysiological investigation of tension headache. *Headache*, 22:173, 1982.
96. Simons, D.J., Day, E., Goodell, H., and Wolff, H.G., Experimental studies on headache: muscles of the scalp and neck as sources of pain. *Assoc. Res. Nerv. Ment. Dis. Proc.*, 23:228, 1943.
97. Robinson, C.A., Cervical spondylosis and muscle contraction headaches, in *Wolff's Headache and Other Head Pain*, 4th ed., Dalessio, D.J. (Ed.) Oxford University Press, New York, 1980, p. 362.
98. Haynes, S.N., Cuevas, J., and Gannon, L.R., The psychophysiological etiology of muscle-contraction headache. *Headache*, 22:122, 1982.

99. Bakal, D.A. and Kaganov, J.A., Muscle contraction and migraine headache: psychophysiologic comparison. *Headache,* 17:208, 1977.
100. Cohen, M.J., Psychological studies of headache: is there a similarity between migraine and muscle contraction headaches? *Headache,* 18:189, 1978.
101. Anderson, C.D. and Franks, R.D., Migraine and tension headache: is there a physiological difference? *Headache,* 21:63, 1981.
102. Pozniak–Patewicz, E., Cephalgic spasm of head and neck muscles. *Headache,* 15:261, 1976.
103. Shoenen, J., Pasqua, V.D., and Sianard-Gainko, J., Multiple clinical and paraclinical analyses of chronic tension-type headache associated or unassociated with disorder of the pericranial muscles. *Cephalalgia,* 11:135, 1991.
104. Langemark, M. and Olesen, J., Pericranial tenderness in tension headache. A blind controlled study. *Cephalalgia,* 7:249, 1987.
105. Langemark, M., Jensen, K., Jensen, T.S., and Olesen, J., Pressure pain thresholds and thermal nociceptive thresholds in chronic tension-type headache. *Pain,* 38:203, 1989.
106. Borgeat, F., Hade, B., Elie, R., and Larouche, L.M., Effects of voluntary muscle tension increases in tension headache. *Headache,* 24:199, 1984.
107. Drummond, P.D., Scalp tenderness and sensitivity to pain in migraine and tension headache. *Headache,* 27:45, 1987.
108. Yang, J.C., Richlin, D., Brand, L., Wagner, J., and Clark, W.C., Thermal sensory decision theory indices and pain threshold in chronic pain patients and healthy volunteers. *Psychol. Med.,* 47:461, 1985.
109. Malow, R.M., Grimm, L., and Olsen, RE., Differences in pain perception between myofascial pain dysfunction and normal subjects: a signal detection analysis. *J. Psychosom. Res.,* 24:303, 1980.
110. Langemark, M. and Jensen, K., Myofascial mechanisms of pain, in *Basic Mechanisms of Headache,* Olesen, J. and Edvinsson, L. (Eds.) Elsevier Science, Amsterdam, 1988, p. 321.
111. Cailliet, R., *Pain: Mechanisms and Management*. F.A. Davis, Philadelphia, 1993, p. 83.
112. Jay, G.W., The autonomic nervous system: anatomy and pharmacology, in *Pain Medicine — A Comprehensive Review,* Raj, P. (Ed.) C.V. Mosby, St. Louis, 1996, pp. 461–465.
113. Langemark, M., Olesen, J., Poulsen, D.P., and Bech, P., Clinical characterization of patients with chronic tension headache. *Headache,* 28:590, 1988.
114. Murphy, A.I. and Lehrer, P.M., Headache versus nonheadache state: a study of electrophysiological and affective changes during muscle contraction headache. *Behav. Med.,* 16:23, 1990.
115. Travell, J. and Rinzler, S.H., The myofascial genesis of pain. *Postgrad. Med.,* 11:425–434, 1952.
116. Travell, J.G. and Simons, D.G., *Myofascial Pain and Dysfunction: The Trigger Point Manual.* Williams & Wilkins, Baltimore, 1983.
117. Jay, G.W., Chronic daily headache and myofascial pain syndromes: pathophysiology and treatment, in *Treating the Headache Patient*, Cady, R.K. and Fox, A.W. (Eds.) Marcel Dekker, New York, 1995, pp. 211–233.
118. Fricton, J.R., Myofascial pain syndrome, in *Advances in Pain Research and Therapy,* Vol. 17, Fricton, J.R. and Awad, E. (Eds.) Raven Press, New York, 1990, p. 107.

119. Fricton, J.R., Kroening, R., Haley, D., and Siegart, R., Myofascial pain syndrome of the head and neck: a review of clinical characteristics of 164 patients. *Oral Surg.*, 60:615, 1985.
120. Philips, C. and Hunter, M., Headache in a psychiatric population. *J. Nerv. Ment. Dis.*, 170:34, 1982.
121. Kudrow, L., Muscle contraction headaches, in *Handbook of Clinical Neurology*, Vol. 48, Rose, F.C. (Ed.) Elsevier Science, Amsterdam, 1986, p. 343.
122. Martin, M.J. and Rome, H.P., Muscle contraction headache: therapeutic aspects. *Res. Clin. Stud. Headache*, 1:205, 1967.
123. Jay, G.W., Grove, R.N., and Grove, K.S., Differentiation of chronic headache from non-headache pain patients using the Millon Clinical Multiaxial Inventory (MCMI). *Headache*, 27:124, 1987.
124. Goldenberg, D.L., Fibromyalgia and chronic fatigue syndrome: are they the same? *J. Musculoskel. Med.*, 7:19, 1990.
125. Mathew, N.T., Glaze, D., and Frost, J., Sleep apnea and other sleep abnormalities in primary headache disorders, in *Migraine: Proceedings of the Fifth International Migraine Symposium*, Rose, C. (Ed.) S. Karger, Basel, 1985, p. 40.
126. Shahota, P.K. and Dexter J.D.S., Sleep and headache syndromes: a clinical review. *Headache*, 30:80, 1990.
127. Drake, M.E., Pakalnis, A., Andrews, J.M., and Bogner, J.F., Nocturnal sleep recording with cassette EEG in chronic headaches. *Headache*, 30:600, 1990.
128. Moldofsky, H., Scariabrick, P., England, R. et al., Musculoskeletal symptoms and non-REM sleep disturbances in patients with fibrositis syndrome and healthy subjects. *Psychosom. Med.*, 37:341, 1975.
129. Goldenberg, D.L., Diagnostic and therapeutic challenges of fibromyalgia. *Hosp. Pract.*, 9:39, 1989.
130. Iansek, R., Heywood, J., Karnaghan, J., and Nalla, J.I., Cervical spondylosis and headaches. *Clin. Exp. Neurol.*, 23e:175, 1987.
131. Forsell, H., Mandibular dysfunction and headache. *Proc. Finn. Dent. Soc.*, 81(Suppl. II):591, 1985.
132. Mikail, M. and Rosen, H., History and etiology of myofascial pain-dysfunction syndrome. *J. Prosthet. Dent.*, 44:438, 1980.
133. Magnusson, T. and Carlsson, G.E., Comparison between two groups of patients in respect to headache and mandibular dysfunction. *Swed. Dent. J.*, 2:85, 1978.
134. Magnusson, T. and Carlsson, G.E., Recurrent headaches in relation to temporomandibular joint pain-dysfunction. *Acta Odontol. Scand.*, 36:333, 1978.
135. Simons, D., Muscular pain syndromes, in *Advances in Pain Research and Therapy*, Vol. 17, Fricton, J.R. and Awad, E. (Eds.) Raven Press, New York, 1990, p. 1.
136. Wolfe, F., Smythe, H.A., Yunas, M.B. et al., The American College of Rheumatology 1990 criteria for the classification of fibromyalgia: a report of the Multicenter Committee. *Arthritis Rheum.*, 33:160, 1990.
137. Campbell, S.M., Clark, S., Tindall, E.A., Forehand, M.E., and Bennett, R.M., Clinical characteristics of fibrositis. 1. A blinded controlled study of symptoms and tender points. *Arthritis Rheum.*, 26:817, 1983.
138. Jay, G.W., Fibromyalgia: a review and hypothesis. *J. Disability*, 1:102, 1991.
139. Bennett, R.M., Myofascial pain syndromes and the fibromyalgia syndrome: a comparative analysis, in *Advances in Pain Research and Therapy*, Vol. 17, Fricton, J.R. and Awad, E. (Eds.) Raven Press, New York, 1990, p. 43.

140. Zidar, J., Backman, E., Bengtsson, A., and Henriksson, K.G., Quantitative EMG and muscle tension and painful muscles in fibromyalgia. *Pain,* 40:249, 1990.
141. Semble, E.L. and Wise, C.M., The fibrositis syndrome, part 1. *Pain Manage.,* Sept/Oct:202, 1988.
142. Rosenhall, U., Johansson, G., and Orndahl, G., Eye motility dysfunction in patients with chronic muscular pain and dysesthesia. *Scand. J. Rehab. Med.,* 19:139, 1987.
143. Henriksson, K.G. and Bengtsson, A., Muscle pain with special reference to primary fibromyalgia (PF), in *Proceedings of the Fifth World Congress on Pain,* Dubner, R., Gebhart, G.F., and Bond, M.R. (Eds.) Elsevier Science, Amsterdam, 1988, p. 232.
144. Vaeroy, H., Zhi–Gai, Q., Morkrid, L. et al., Altered sympathetic nervous system response in patients with fibromyalgia (fibrositis syndrome). *J. Rheumatol.,* 16:1460, 1989.
145. Jay, G.W., Myofascial Mechanisms in the Etiology of Chronic Daily Headache: Two Syndromes, One Entity? Paper presented at the 32d Annual Meeting of the American Association for the Study of Headache, Los Angeles, June, 1990.
146. Olesen, J., Clinical characterization of tension headache, in *Basic Mechanisms of Headache,* Olesen, J. and Edvinsson, L. (Eds.) Elsevier Science, Amsterdam, 1988, p. 9.
147. Cohen, M.J., Psychophysiological studies of headache: is there similarity between migraine and muscle contraction headaches? *Headache,* 18:189, 1978.
148. Tfelt-Hansen, P., Lous, I., and Olesen, J., Prevalence and significance of muscle tenderness during common migraine attacks. *Headache,* 21:49, 1981.
149. Olesen, J., Some clinical features of the acute migraine attack. An analysis of 750 patients. *Headache,* 18:268, 1978.
150. Ellertsen, B., Norby, H., and Sjaastad, O., Psychophysiological response patterns in tension headache: effects of tricyclic antidepressants. *Cephalalgia,* 7:55, 1987.
151. Haynes, S.N., Muscle contraction headache: a psychophysiological perspective, in *Psychosomatic Disorders: A Psychophysiologyical Approach to Etiology and Treatment,* Haynes, S.N. and Gannon, L.R. (Eds.) Praeger Press, New York, 1981.
152. Tunis, M.M. and Wolff, H.G., Studies on headache: cranial artery vasoconstriction and muscle contraction headache. *Arch. Neurol. Psychiatry,* 71:425, 1954.
153. Mikamo, K., Takeshima, T., and Takahashi, K., Cardiovascular sympathetic hypofunction in muscle contraction headache and migraine. *Headache,* 29:86, 1989.
154. Covelli, V. and Ferrannini, E., Neurophysiologic findings in headache patients. Psychogalvanic reflex investigation in migraineurs and tension headache patients. *Acta Neurol.,* 9:354, 1987.
155. Takeshima, T., Takao, Y., and Takahashi, K., Pupillary sympathetic hypofunction and asymmetry in muscle contraction headache. *Cephalalgia,* 7:257, 1987.
156. Shimomura, T. and Takahashi, K., Pupillary functional asymmetry in patients with muscle contraction headache. *Cephalalgia,* 6:141, 1986.
157. Drummond, P.D., A quantitative assessment of photophobia in migraine and tension headache. *Headache,* 26:465, 1986.
158. Hanington, E., Jones, R.J., Amess, J.A.L., and Wachowicz, B., Migraine: a platelet disorder. *Lancet,* ii:720, 1981.

159. D'Andrea, G., Toledo, M., Cortelazzo, S., and Milone, F.F., Platelet activity in migraine. *Headache,* 22:207, 1982.
160. Rolf, L.H., Wiele, G., and Brune, G.G., 5-Hydroxytryptamine in platelets of patients with muscle contraction headache. *Headache,* 21:10, 1981.
161. Basbaum, A.I. and Fields, H.L., Endogenous pain control systems: brainstem spinal pathways and endorphin circuitry. *Annu. Rev. Neurosci.,* 7:309, 1984.
162. Andersen, E. and Dafny, N., An ascending serotonergic pain modulation pathway from the dorsal raphe nucleus to the parafascicularis nucleus of the thalamus. *Brain Res.,* 269:57, 1983.
163. Raskin, N.H., On the origin of head pain. *Headache,* 28:254, 1988.
164. Raskin, N.H., *Headache,* 2nd ed. Churchill Livingstone, New York, 1988.
165. Fields, H.L., Sources of variability in the sensation of pain. *Pain,* 33:195, 1988.
166. Wall, P.D., Stability and instability of central pain mechanisms, in *Proceedings of the Fifth World Conference on Pain.* Dubner, R. and Bond, M.R. (Eds.) Elsevier Science, Amsterdam, 1988, p. 13.
167. Terenius, L., Endorphins and modulation of pain, in *Advances in Neurology,* Vol. 33, Critchley, M., Friedman, A.P., Gorini, S., Sicuteri, F. et al. (Eds.) Raven Press, New York, 1982, p. 59.
168. Sicuteri, F., Natural opiods in migraine, in *Advances in Neurology,* Vol. 33, Critchley, M., Friedman, A.P., Gorini, S., Sicuteri, F. et al. (Eds.) Raven Press, New York, 1982, p. 65.
169. Sicuteri, F., Spillantini, M.G., and Fanciullacci, M., "Enkephalinase" in migraine and opiate addiction, in *Migraine: Proceedings of the Fifth International Migraine Symposium,* Rose, C. (Ed.) S. Karger, Basel, 1985, p. 86.
170. Mosnaim, A.D., Diamond, S., Wolf, M.E. et al., Endogenous opiod-like peptides in headache: an overview. *Headache,* 29:368, 1989.
171. Genazzani, A.R., Nappi, G., Facchinetti, F. et al., Progressive impairment of CSF B-EP levels in migraine sufferers. *Pain,* 18:127, 1984.
172. Facchinetti, F. and Genazzani, A.R., Opiods in cerebrospinal fluid and blood of headache sufferers, in *Basic Mechanisms of Headache,* Olesen, J. and Edvinsson, L. (Eds.) Elsevier Science, Amsterdam, 1988, p. 261.
173. Nappi, G., Gacchinetti, G., Legnante, G. et al., Impairment of the Central and Peripheral Opiod System in Headache. Paper presented at the Fourth International Migraine Trust Symposium, London, 1982.
174. Gawel, M., Fettes, I., Kuzniak, S., and Edmeads, J., Endorphin levels in headache syndromes, in *Migraine: Proceedings of the Fifth International Migraine Symposium,* Rose, C. (Ed.) S. Karger, Basel, 1985, p. 66.
175. Bella, D.D., Carenzi, A., Casacci, F. et al., Endorphins in the pathogenesis of headache, in *Advances in Neurology,* Vol. 33, Critchley, M., Friedman, A.P., Gorini, S., Sicuteri, F. et al (Eds.) Raven Press, New York, 1982, p. 75.
176. Pletsher, A., Affolter, H., Cesuro, A.M., Ezne, P., and Muller, K., Blood platelets as a model for neurons: similarities of the 5-hydroxytryptamine system, in Schlessberger, H.G., Kocheau, W., Linzen, B., and Steinbast, H. (Eds.) Walter de Gzuyter, Berlin, 1984, p. 231.
177. Giacovazzo, M., Bernoni, R.M., Di Sabato, F., and Martelletti, P., Impairment of 5HT binding to lymphocytes and monocytes from tension-type headache patients. *Headache,* 30: 20, 1990.
178. Shimomura, T. and Takahashi, K., Alteration of platelet serotonin in patients with chronic tension-type headache during cold pressor test. *Headache,* 30:581, 1990.

179. Pernow, B., Substance P. *Pharmacol Rev.*, 35:85, 1983.
180. Almay, B.G.L., Johansson, F., von Knorring, L. et al., Substance P in CSF of patients with chronic pain syndromes. *Pain*, 33:3, 1988.
181. Kowa, H., Shimomura, T., and Takahashi, K., Platelet gamma-amino butyric acid levels in migraine and tension-type headache. *Headache*, 32:229, 1992.
182. Takeshima, T., Takao, Y., Urakami, K. et al., Muscle contraction headache and migraine. Platelet activation and plasma norepinephrine during the cold pressor test. *Cephalalgia*, 9:7, 1989.
183. Sicuteri, F., Nicolodi, M., and Fusco, B.M., Abnormal sensitivity to neurotransmitter agonists, antagonists and neurotransmitter releasers, in *Basic Mechanisms of Headache*, Olesen, J. and Edvinsson, L. (Eds.) Elsevier Science, Amsterdam, 1988, p. 275.
184. Jay, G.W., Brunson, J., and Branson, S.J., The effectiveness of physical therapy in the treatment of chronic daily headaches. *Headache*, 29:156, 1989.
185. Fordyce, W.E., Behavioral conditioning concepts in chronic pain, in *Advances in Pain Research and Therapy*, Vol. 5, Bonica, J.J., Lindblom, U., and Iggo, A. (Eds.) Raven Press, New York, 1983.
186. Lazarus, R.S. and Folkman, S., *Stress, Appraisal and Coping*. Springer-Verlag, New York, 1984.
187. Kanner, A.D., Coyne, N.C., Schaefer, C., Lazarus, R.S., Comparison of two modes of stress measurement: daily hassles and uplifts versus major life events. *J. Behav. Med.*, 4:1–39, 1981.
188. Rose, C.L. and Gawel, M., What brings on a migraine attack?, in *Migraine: The Facts*, Oxford University Press, London, 1979, p. 42.
189. Selye, H., *The Stress of Life*. McGraw-Hill, New York, 1976, p. 412.
190. Wolff, H.G., *Headache and Other Head Pain*, 2nd ed. Oxford University Press, New York, 1963.
191. Jay, G.W., Grove, R.N., and Grove, K.S., Differentiation of chronic headache from non-headache pain patients using the Millon Clinical Multiaxial Inventory (MCMI). *Headache*, 27:124–129, 1987.
192. Derogatis, L.R., *R-Version Manual–1: Scoring Administration and Procedures for the SCL–90*. Johns Hopkins University Press, Baltimore, 1977.
193. Ellertson, B., Troland, K., and Klove, H., MMPI profiles in migraine before and after biofeedback treatment. *Cephalalgia*, 7:101–108, 1987.
194. Nicholson, N.L., Blanchard, E.B., and Appelbaum, K.A., Two studies of the occurrence of psychophysiological symptoms in chronic headache patients. *Behav. Res. Ther.*, 28:195–203, 1990.
195. Rapport, N.B., McAnulty, D.P., Waggoner, C.D., and Brantley, P.J., Cluster analysis of Minnesota Multiphasic Personality Inventory (MMPI) profiles in a chronic headache population. *J. Behav. Med.*, 10:49–60, 1987.
196. Kinder, B.N., Curtiss, G., and Kalichman, S., Cluster analyses of headache patient MMPI scores: a cross validation. *Psychol. Assess.*, 3:226–231, 1991.
197. Robinson, M.E., Geisser, M.E., Dieter, J.N., and Swerdlow, B., The relationship between MMPI cluster membership and diagnostic category in headache patients. *Headache*, 31:111–115, 1991.
198. Cram, J.R., EMG biofeedback and the treatment of tension headaches: a systematic analysis of treatment components. *Behav. Ther.*, 11:699–710, 1980.

199. Sovak, M., Kunzel, M., Sternbach, R., and Dalessio, D.J., Mechanisms of the biofeedback therapy of migraine: volitional manipulation of the psychophysiological background. *Headache,* 21:89–92, 1981.
200. Mosley, T.H., Penzien, D.B., Johnson, C.A., Brantley, P.J., Wittrock, D.A. et al., Time–series analysis of stress and headache. *Cephalalgia,* 11:306–307, 1991.
201. Levor, R.M., Cohen, M.J., Naliboff, B.K., McArthur, D., and Heuser, G., Psychosocial precursors and correlates of migraine headache. *J. Consult. Clin. Psychol.,* 54:347–353, 1986.
202. Sorbi, M. and Tellgen, B., Stress coping in migraine. *Soc. Sci. Med.,* 26:351–358, 1988.
203. Miznener, D., Thomas, M., and Billings, R., Cognitive changes of migraineurs receiving biofeedback training. *Headache,* 28:339–343, 1988.
204. Wallston, K.A., Wallston, B.S., and De Villis, R., Development of the multidimensional health locus of control (MHLC) scales. *Health Educ. Monogr.,* 6:160–170, 1978.
205. Martin, N., Holroyd, K.A., and Penzien, D.B., The headache specific locus of control scale: adaptation to recurrent headaches. *Headache,* 30:729–734, 1990.
206. Hudzynski, L.G. and Levenson, H., Biofeedback behavioral treatment of headache with locus of control pain analysis: a 20-month retrospective study. *Headache,* 25:380–386, 1985.
207. Jay, G.W., Goka, R.S., Arakaki, A.H., Mild traumatic brain injury: review of clinical data and appropriate evaluation and treatment. *J. Insur. Med.,* 27:62–282, 1996.
208. Denny-Brown, D. and Russell, W.R., Experimental cerebral concussion. *Brain,* 64:93, 1941.
209. Kay, T., Harrington, D.E. et al., Definition of mild traumatic brain injury. *J. Head Trauma Rehabil.,* 8(3):86–87, 1993.
210. Zasler, N.D., Neuromedical diagnosis and management of post–concussive disorders. *Phys. Med. Rehabil. State Art Rev.,* 6:3–67, 1992.
211. Oppenheimer, D.R., Microscopic lesions in the brain following head injury. *J. Neurol. Neurosurg. Psychiatry,* 31:299–306, 1968.
212. Boll, T.J. and Barth, J., Mild head injury. *Psychiatr. Dev.,* 1(3):509–513, 1983.
213. Pilz, P., Axonal injury in head injury. *Acta Neurochyir.,* 32:119–26, 1983.
214. Peerless, S. and Rewcastle, N., Shear injuries of the brain. *Can. Med. Assoc. J.,* 96:577–582, 1967.
215. Taylor, A.R. and Bell, T.K., Slowing of cerebral circulation after concussional head injury. *Lancet,* 2:178–180, 1966.
216. Povlishock, J.T., Becker, D.P., Cheng, C.L.Y., and Vaughn, G.W., Axonal change in minor head injury. *J. Neuropathol. Exp. Neurol.,* 42:225–242, 1983.
217. Stritch, S.J., Shearing of nerve fibers as a cause of brain injury due to head injury: a pathological study of twenty cases. Lancet, ii:443–448, 1961.
218. Gennarelli, T.A., Mechanisms of brain injury. *J. Emerg. Med.,* 11(Suppl. 1): 5–11, 1993.
219. Hayes, R.L., Lyeth, B.G., and Jenkins, L.W., Neurochemical mechanisms of mild and moderate head injury: implications for treatment, in *Mild Head Injury,* Levin, H.S., Eisenberg, H.M., and Benton, A.L. (Eds.) Oxford University Press, New York, 1989, pp. 54–79.

220. Gorman, L.K., Fu, K., Hovda, K. et al., Analysis of acetylcholine release following concussive brain injury in the rat. *J. Neurotrauma,* 6:203, 1989.
221. Smith, D.H., Okiyama, K., Thomas, M.J., and McIntosh, T.K., An NMDA receptor associated glycine site antagonist attenuates memory loss after experimental brain injury. *Soc. Neurosci. Abstr.,* 16:779, 1990.
222. Faden, A.I., Demediuk, P., Panter, S.S., and Vink, R., The role of excitatory amino acids and NMDA receptors in traumatic brain injury. *Science,* 244:798–800, 1989.
223. Erb, D.E. and Povlishock, J.T., Neuroplasticity following traumatic brain injury: a study of GABAnergic terminal loss and recovery in the cat dorsal lateral vestibular nucleus. *Exp. Brain Res.,* 83:253–267, 1991.
224. Povlishock, J.T. and Lyeth, B.G., Traumatically induced blood-brain barrier disruption: a conduit for the passage of circulating excitatory neurotransmitters. *Soc. Neurosci. Abstr.,* 15:1113, 1989
225. Bohnen, N. and Jolles, J., Neurobehavioral aspects of postconcussive symptoms after mild head injury. *J. Nerv. Ment. Dis.,* 180(11):683–692, 1992.
226. Bohnen, N., Twijnstra, A., and Jolles, J., Post-traumatic and emotional symptoms in different subgroups of patients with mild head injury. *Brain Inj.,* 6(6):481–487, 1992.
227. Szymanski, H.V. and Linn, R., A review of the postconcussion syndrome. *Int. J. Psychiatr. Med.,* 22(4):357–375. 1992.
228. Jakobsen, J., Baadsgaard, S.E., Thomsen, S., and Henriksen, P.B., Prediction of post-concussional sequelae by reaction time test. *Acta Neurol. Scand.,* 75(5):341–345, 1987.
229. Alexander, M.P., Mild traumatic brain injury: pathophysiology, natural history and clinical management. *Neurology,* 45:1253–1260, 1995.
230. Rutherford, W.H., Merrett, J.D., and McDonald, J.R., Symptoms at one year following concussion from minor head injuries. *Injury,* 10:225–230, 1978–1979.
231. McLean, A., Temkin, N.R., Dikmen, S. et al., The behavioral sequelae of head injury. *J. Clin. Neuropsychol.,* 5:361–376, 1983.
232. Evans, R.W., Mild traumatic brain injury. *Phys. Med. Rehabil. Clin. N. Am.,* 3(2):427–439, 1992.
233. Berrol, S., Terminology of post-concussive syndrome. *Phys. Med. Rehabil. State Art Rev.,* 6(1):1–8, 1992.
234. Stuss, D.T., Ely, P., Hugenholtz, H. et al., Subtle neuropsychological deficits in patients with good recovery after closed head injury. *Neurosurgery,* 17:41–47, 1985.
235. Jones, J.H., Viola, S.L., LaBan, M.M., Schynoll, W.G., and Krome, R.L., The incidence of post minor traumatic brain injury syndrome: a retrospective survey of treating physicians. *Arch. Phys. Med. Rehabil.,* 73(2):145–146, 1992.
236. Katz, R.T. and DeLuca, J., Sequelae of minor traumatic brain injury. *Am. Fam. Physician,* 46(5):1491–1498, 1992.
237. Wrightson, P. and Gronwall, D., Time off work and symptoms after minor head injury. *Injury,* 12(6):445–454, 1981.
238. Leininger, B.E., Gramling, S.E., Farrell, A.D., Kreutzer, J.S., and Peck, E.A., Neuropsychological deficits in symptomatic minor head injury patients after concussion and mild concussion. *J. Neurol. Neurosurg. Psychiatry,* 53(4): 293–296, 1990.

239. Harrington, D.E., Malec, J., Cicerone, K., and Katz, H.T., Current perceptions of rehabilitation professionals towards mild traumatic brain injury. *Arch. Phys. Med. Rehabil.*, 74(6):579–586, 1993.
240. Middelboe, T., Anderson, H.S., Birket-Smith, M., and Friis, M.L., Minor head injury: impact on general health after 1 year. A prospective follow-up study. *Acta Neurol. Scand.*, 85(1):5–9, 1992.
241. Alexander, M.P., Neuropsychiatric correlates of persistent postconcussive syndrome. *J. Head Trauma Rehabil.*, 7(2):60–69, 1992.
242. Radanov, B.P., Di Stefano, G., Schnidrig, A. et al., Role of psychosocial stress in recovery from common whiplash. *Lancet*, 338:712–715, 1991.
243. Ettlin, T.M., Kischka, U., Reichmann, S. et al., Cerebral symptoms after whiplash injury of the neck: a prospective clinical and neuropsychological study of whiplash injury. *J. Neurol. Neurosurg. Psychiatry*, 55:943–948, 1993.
244. Schoenhuber, R. and Gentilini, M., Anxiety and depression after mild head injury: a case control study. *J. Neurol. Neurosurg. Psychiatry*, 51:722–724, 1988.
245. Jay, G.W., Chronic tension-type headache, in *Office Practice of Neurology*, Samuels, M.A., Feske, S., Mesulam, M.M. et al. (Eds.) Churchill Livingstone, New York, 1996, pp. 1118–1123.
246. Jay, G.W., Chronic daily headache: pathophysiology and treatment. *Pain Digest*, 4:257–268, 1994.
247. Haas, D.C., Pineda, G.S., Lourie, H. et al., Juvenile head trauma syndromes and their relationship to migraine. *Arch. Neurol.*, 32:727–730, 1975.
248. Bennet, E.R., Migraine precipitated by head trauma in wrestling. *Am. J. Sports Med.*, 8:202–205, 1974.
249. Behrman, S., Migraine as a sequela of blunt head injury. *Injury*, 9:74–76, 1977.
250. Jacobson, S.A., Mechanism of the sequelae of minor craniocervical trauma, in *Late Effects of Head Injury*, Walker, A.E., Caveness, W.F., and Critchley, M., (Eds.) Charles C Thomas, Springfield, IL, 1969, pp. 33–45.
251. Evans, R,W., The postconcussion syndrome and the sequelae of mild head injury. *Neurol. Clin.*, 10(4):815–847, 1992
252. Cicerone, K.D., Psychological management of post-concussive disorders. *Phys. Med. Rehabil. State Art Rev.*, 6(1):129–141, 1992.
253. Elkind, A.H., Headache and facial pain associated with head injury. *Otolaryngol. Clin. North Am.*, 22(6):1251–1271, 1989.
254. Merskey, H. and Woodford, J.M., Psychiatric sequelae after minor head injury. *Brain*, 95:521–528, 1972.
255. Watson, C.P.N., Deck, J.H., Morshead, C., Van Der Kooy, D., and Evans, R.J., Postherpetic neuralgia: further post-mortem studies of cases with and without pain. *Pain*, 44:105–117, 1991.
256. Mathew, N.T. and Chandy, J., Painful ophthalmoplegia. *J. Neurol. Sci.*, 11:243–256, 1970.
257. Portenoy, R.K., Duma, C., and Foley, K.M., Acute herpetic and postherpetic neuralgia: clinical review and current management. *Ann. Neurol.*, 20:651–664, 1986.
258. Hatangdi, V.S., Boas, R.A., and Richards, E.G., Postherpetic neuralgia: management with antiepileptic and tricyclic drugs, in *Advances in Pain Research and Therapy*, Vol. 1, Bonica, J.J. and Albe-Fessard, D. (Eds.) Raven Press, New York, 1976, pp. 583–587.

259. Rushton, J.G., Stevens, C., and Miller, R.H., Glossopharyngeal (vagoglossopharyngeal) neuralgia. *Arch. Neurol.*, 38:201–205, 1981.
260. Raskin, N.H. and Prusiner, S., Carotidynia. *Neurology*, 27:43–46, 1977
261. Vijayan, N. and Watson, C., Raeder's syndrome, pericarotid syndrome and carotidynia, in *Handbook of Clinical Neurology*. Vol. 4(48). *Headache*, Vinken, P.J. and Bruyn, G.W. (Eds.) Elsevier, Amsterdam, 1986, pp. 329–341.
262. Roseman, D.M., Carotidynia. *N.Y. State J. Med.*, 63:2651–2653, 1963.
263. Lovshin, L.L., Vascular neck pain: a common syndrome seldom recognized. *Cleveland Clin. A.*, 27:5–13, 1960.
264. Roseman, D.M., Carotidynia: a distinct syndrome. *Arch. Otolaryngol.*, 85:81–84, 1967.
265. Pearce, H.E. and Hinshaw, J.R., Bilateral arteritis simulating carotid body tumors. *Surg. Gynecol. Obstetr.*, 103:263–266, 1956.
266. Hilger, J.A., Carotid pain. *Laryngoscope*, 59:829–838, 1949.
267. Bogduk, N., An anatomical basis for neck tongue syndrome. *J. Neurol. Neurosurg. Psychiatry*, 44:202–208, 1981.
268. Lance, J.W. and Anthony, M., Neck-tongue syndrome on sudden turning of the head. *J. Neurol. Neurosurg. Psychiatry*, 43:97–101, 1980.
269. Bertoft, E.S. and Westerberg, C.E., Further observations on the neck-tongue syndrome. *Cephalalgia*, 5(Suppl. 3):312–313, 1985.
270. Fortin, C.J. and Biller, J., Neck-tongue syndrome. *Headache*, 25:255–258, 1985.
271. Elisevich, K., Stratford, J., Bray, G., and Finlayson, M., Neck-tongue syndrome: operative management. *J. Neurol. Neurosurg. Psychiatry*, 47:407–409, 1984.
272. Hunt, W.E., Tolosa-Hunt syndrome: one cause of painful ophthalmoplegia. *J. Neurosurg.*, 44:544–549, 1976.
273. Mathew, N.T. and Chandy, J., Painful ophthalmoplegia. *J. Neurol. Sci.*, 11:243–256, 1970.
274. Hunt, W.E., Meagher, J,N., Lefever, H.E., and Zeman, W., Painful ophthalmoplegia: its relation to indolent inflammation of the cavernous sinus. *Neurology*, 11:56–62, 1961.
275. Takeoka, T., Gotoh, F., Fukuchi, V., and Inagaki, Y., Tolosa-Hunt syndrome: arteriographic evidence of improvement in carotid narrowing. *Arch. Neurol.*, 35:219–223, 1978.
276. Hannerz, J., Recurrent Tolosa-Hunt syndrome. *Cephalalgia*, 12:45–51, 1992.
277. Raeder, J.G., "Paratrigeminal" paralysis of oculo-pupillary sympathetic. *Brain*, 47:149–158, 1924.
278. Vijayan, N. and Watson, C., Pericarotid syndrome. *Headache*, 18:244–254, 1978.
279. Tasker, R.R., Carvalho, G., and Dostrovsky, J.O., The history of central pain syndromes, with observations concerning pathophysiology and treatment, in *Pain and Central Nervous System Disease: The Central Pain Syndromes*, Casey, K.L. (Ed.) Raven Press, New York, 1991, pp. 31–58.
280. Pagni, C.A., Central pain due to spinal cord and brainstem damage, in *Textbook of Pain*, Wall, P.D. and Melzack, R.D. (Eds.) Churchill Livingstone, New York, 1989, pp. 634–655.
281. Lenz, F.A., The thalamus and central pain syndromes: human and animal studies, in *Pain and Central Nervous System Disease: The Central Pain Syndromes*, Casey, K.L. (Ed.) Raven Press, New York, 1991, pp. 171–182.

282. Tasker, R.R., Pain resulting from central nervous system pathology (central pain), in Bonica, J.J. (Ed.) *The Management of Pain*, 2nd ed., Lea & Febiger, Philadelphia, 1990, pp. 264–280.
283. Cesaro, P., Mann, M.W., Moretti, J.L., Defer, G., Roualdes, B., Nguyen, J.P., and Degos, J.D., Central pain and thalamic hyperactivity: a single photon emission computerized tomographic study. *Pain*, 47:329–336, 1991.
284. Dubner R., Neuronal plasticity and pain following peripheral tissue inflammation or nerve injury, in *Proceedings of the Sixth World Congress on Pain*, Bond, M.R., Charlton, J., and Woolf, C.J. (Eds.) Elsevier, Amsterdam, 1991, pp. 343–347.
285. Leijon, G. and Boivie, J., Central post-stroke pain: a controlled trial of amitriptyline and carbamazepine. *Pain*, 36:27–36, 1989.
286. Budd, K., The use of the opiate antagonist, naloxone, in the treatment of intractable pain. *Neuropeptides*, 5:419–422, 1985.
287. Loh, L., Nathan, P.W., and Schott, G.D., Pain due to lesions of the central nervous system removed by sympathetic block. *Br. Med. J.*, 282:1026–1028, 1981.
288. Albrecht, K. and Krump, J., Diagnose, Differentialdiagnose und Behandlungsmoglichkeiten-der Trigeminusyneuralgie. *Muenchen. Med. Wschr.*, 96:985–990, 1954.
289. White, J.C. and Sweet, W.H., *Pain and the Neurosurgeon., A Forty-Year Experience*. Charles C Thomas, Springfield, IL, 1969.
290. Fothergill, J., Of a painful affection of the face: medical observations and inquiries by a society of physicians. *London*, 5:129–142, 1773.
291. Jannetta, P.J., Surgical treatment microvascular decompression, in *Trigeminal Neuralgia Current Concepts Regarding Pathogenesis and Treatment*, Fromm, G.H. and Sessle, B.J. (Eds.) Butterworth–Heinemann, Boston, 1991, pp. 145–157.
292. Terrence, C.F., Costa, R., and Fromm, G.H., An unusual case of paroxysmal face pain. *J. Neurol.*, 221:73–76, 1979.
293. Fromm, G.H., Pathophysiology of trigeminal neuralgia, in *Trigeminal Neuralgia Current Concepts Regarding Pathogenesis and Treatment*, Fromm, G.H. and Sessle, B.J. (Eds.) Butterworth–Heinemann, Boston, 1991, pp. 131–140.
294. Fromm, G.H., Neuralgia of the face and oral cavity. *Pain Dig.*, 1:67–77, 1991.
295. Blom, S., Trigeminal neuralgia: its treatment with a new anticonvulsant drug (G32883). *Lancet*, 1:839–840, 1962.
296. Fromm, G.H., Terrence, C.F., Chattha, A.S., and Glass, J.D., Baclofen in trigeminal neuralgia: its effect on the spinal trigeminal nucleus. A pilot study. *Arch. Neurol.*, 37:768–781, 1980.
297. Browne, L., Radiofrequency lesioning of the trigeminal ganglion for the treatment of trigeminal neuralgia. *Irish Med. J.*, 78:68–71, 1985.
298. Nugent, G.R., Surgical treatment: radiofrequency gangliolysis and rhizotomy, in *Trigeminal Neuralgia Current Concepts Regarding Pathogenesis and Treatment*, Fromm, G.H. and Sessle, B.J. (Eds.) Butterworth–Heinemann, Boston, 1991, pp. 159–184.
299. Hakanson, S., Surgical treatment: retrogassarian glycerol injection, in *Trigeminal Neuralgia Current Concepts Regarding Pathogenesis and Treatment*, Fromm, G.H. and Sessle, B.J. (Eds.) Butterworth–Heinemann, Boston, 1991, pp. 185–204.

300. Gelb, H. and Bernstein, I., Clinical evaluation of 200 patients with temporomandibular joint syndrome. *J. Prosth. Dent.*, 49:234–243, 1983.
301. Merrill, R.L. and Graff-Radford, S.B., Trigeminal neuralgia: how to rule out the wrong treatment. *J. Am. Dent. Assoc.*, 123:63–68, 1992.
302. Court, J.E. and Kase, C.S., Treatment of tic douloureux with a new anticonvulsant (clonazepam). *J. Neurol. Neurosurg. Psychiatry*, 39:297–299, 1976.
303. Pujol, M., *Essai sue la Maladie de la Face Nomme le Tic Doulourex.* Theophile Barrois, Paris, 1787.
304. Solomon, S. and Lipton, R.B., Atypical facial pain: a review. *Semin. Neurol.*, 8:332–338, 1988.
305. Solomon, S. and Lipton, R.B., Facial pain, *Neurol. Clin.*, 8:913–928, 1990.
306. Dalessio, D.J., The major neuralgias, postinfectious neuritis, intractable pain and atypical facial pain, in *Wolff's Headache and Other Head Pain*. Oxford University Press, New York, 1980.
307. Dworkin, S.F. and Burgess, J.A., Orofacial pain of psychogenic origin: current concepts and classification. *J. Am. Dent. Assoc.*, 115:565–571, 1987.
308. Lehmann, H.J. and Buchholz, G., Atypical facial neuralgia or depressive facial pain. Diagnostic aspects of a well-demarcated form of masked depression. *Fortschr. Neurol. Psychiatr.*, 54:154–157, 1986.
309. McNeill, C. (Ed.): *Craniomandibular Disorders: Guidelines for Evaluation, Diagnosis and Management*, 2nd ed. Quintessence, Chicago, 1992.
310. Agerberg, D. and Carlsson, G.E., Late results of treatment of functional disorders of the masticatory system. A follow-up by questionnaire. *J. Oral Rehab.*, 1:309–316, 1974.
311. Forssell, H., Kirveskari, P., and Kangasniemi, P., Distinguishing between headaches responsive and irresponsive to treatment of mandibular dysfunction. *Proc. Finn. Dent. Soc.*, 82:219–222, 1986.
312. Magnusson, T. and Carlsson, G.E., Changes in recurrent headache and mandibular dysfunction after various types of dental treatment. *Acta Odont. Scand.*, 38:311–320, 1980.
313. Schiffman, E., Fricton, J.R., Haley, D., and Shapiro, B.L., The prevalence and treatment needs of subjects with temporomandibular disorders. *J. Am. Dent. Assoc.*, 120:295–304, 1989.
314. Berlin, R. and Dressner, L., Bruxism and chronic headache. *Lancet*, 2:289–291, 1960.
315. Forssell, H., Kirveskari, P., and Kangasniemi, P., Changes in headache after treatment of mandibular dysfunction. *Cephalalgia*, 5:229–236, 1985.
316. Gelb, H. and Tarte, J., A two-year clinical dental evaluation of 200 cases of chronic headache: the cranio-cervical mandibular syndrome. *J. Am. Dent. Assoc.*, 91:1230–1236, 1975.
317. Forsell, H. and Kangasniemi, P., Mandibular dysfunction in patients with migraine. *Proc. Finn. Dent. Soc.*, 80:211–216, 1986.
318. Lance, J.W., *Mechanism and Management of Headache*, 4th ed. Butterworth & Co., Ltd., London, 1982.
319. Hardebo, J.E., An association between cluster headache and herpes simplex. *N. Engl. J. Med.*, 314–316, 1986.
320. Tunkel, A.R., Wispelwey, B., and Scheld, W.M., Bacterial meningitis: recent advances in pathophysiology and treatment. *Ann. Intern. Med.*, 112:610–613, 1990.

321. Anzola, G.P., Dalla Bolta, G., and Balestrieri, G., Headache in patients with systemic lupus erythematosus: clinical and telethermographic findings. *Arch. Neurol.*, 45:1061–1062, 1988.
322. Caskey, W.H. and Spierings, E.L.H., Headache and heartache. *Headache*, 18:240–243, 1978.
323. Loeb, C. and Gandolfo, C., Headache in ischemic cerebrovascular disease. *Neurology*, 37:1266, 1987.
324. Edmeads, J., Headaches in cerebrovascular disease. *Postgrad. Med.*, 81:191–198, 1987.
325. Iansek, R., Cervical spondylosis and headaches. *Clin. Exp. Neurol.*, May:175–178, 1982.
326. Schumacher, G.A. and Wolff, H.G., Experimental studies on headache. *Arch. Neurol. Psychiatry*, 45:199–214, 1941.
327. Ray, B.S. and Wolff, H.G., Experimental studies on headache. Pain sensitive structures of the head and their significance in headache. *Arch. Surg.*, 41:813–856, 1940.
328. Symonds, C., Cough headache. *Brain*, 79:557–568, 1956.
329. Rooke, E.D., Benign exertional headache. *Med. Clin. North Am.*, 52:801–808, 1968.
330. Cameron, M.E., Headaches in relation to the eyes. *Med. J. Aust.*, 1:292–294, 1976.
331. Schultz, D.R., Occipital neuralgia. *J. Am. Osteopathic Assoc.*, 76:335–342, 1977.
332. Hunter, C.R. and Mayfield, F.H., Role of the upper cervical roots in the production of pain in the head. *Am. J. Surg.*, 78:743–749, 1949.
333. Hammond, S.R. and Danta, G., Occipital neuralgia. *Clin. Exp. Neurol.*, 15:258–270, 1978.
334. Cox, C.L. and Cocks, G.R., Occipital neuralgia. *J. Med. Assoc. ALA*, January:23–32, 1979.
335. Bogduk, N., The anatomy of occipital neuralgia. *Clin. Exp. Neurol.*, 17:167–184, 1980.
336. Bogduk, N., The clinical anatomy of the cervical dorsal rami. *Spine*, 7:319–330, 1982.
337. Vital, J.M., Grenier, F., Dautheribes, M., Baspeyre, H., Lavignolle, B., and Senegas, J., An anatomic and dynamic study of the greater occipital nerve (n. of Arnold). *Surg. Radiol. Anat.*, 11:205–210, 1989.
338. Ehni, G. and Benner, B.L., Occipital neuralgia and the C_{1-2} arthrosis syndrome. *J. Neurosurg.*, 61:961–965, 1984.
339. Cook, N., Cryosurgery of headache. *Res. Clin. Stud. Headache*, 5:86–101, 1978.
340. Sluder, G., The role of sphenopalatine (or Meckel's) ganglion in nasal headaches. *N.Y. Med. J.*, 87:989, 1908.
341. Vail, H.H., Vidian neuralgia. *Ann. Otol.*, 41:837–856, 1932.
342. Edmeads, J., The cervical spine and headache. *Neurology*, 38:1874–1878, 1988.
343. Kerr, F.W.L., A mechanism to account for frontal headaches in cases of posterior fossa tumors. *J. Neurosurg.*, 18:605–609, 1961.
344. Khurana, R., Headache spectrum in Arnold-Chiari malformation. *Headache*, 31:151–155, 1991.
345. Hawkins, G.W., Flexion and extension injuries of the cervico-capital joints. *Clin. Orthop.*, 24:22–33, 1962.

346. Weiss, H.D., Stern, B.J., and Goldberg, J., Post-traumatic migraine: chronic migraine precipitated by minor head or neck trauma. *Headache,* 31:451–456, 1991.
347. Sjaastad, O., Fredriksen, T.A., and Pfaffenrath, V., Cervicogenic headache: diagnostic criteria. *Headache,* 30:725–726, 1990.
348. Vernon, H., Vertebrogenic headache, in *Upper Cervical Syndrome: Chiropractic Diagnosis and Treatment,* Vernon, H. (Ed.) Williams & Wilkins, Baltimore, 1988, pp. 152–188.
349. Sjaastad, O. and Bovim, G., Cervicogenic headache: the differentiation from common migraine. An overview. *Func. Neurol.,* 6:93–100, 1991
350. Greenman, P.E., Manipulation and mobilization, in *Headache: Diagnosis and Treatment,* Tollison, C.D. and Kunkel, R.S. (Eds.) Williams & Wilkins, Baltimore, 1993, pp. 347–355.
351. Dvorak, J., Dvorak, V., and Schneider, W., *Manual Medicine.* Springer–Verlag, Berlin, 1984.
352. Solomon, S., Elkind, A., Freitag, F.G., Gallagher, R.M., Moore, K. et al., Safety and efficacy of cranial electrotherapy in the treatment of tension headache. *Headache,* 29:445–450, 1989.
353. Hoyt, W.H., Shaffer, F., Bard, D.A., Benesler, J.S., Blankenhorn, G.D. et al., Osteopathic manipulation in the treatment of muscle-contraction headache. *J. Am. Osteopath. Assoc.,* 78:322–325, 1979.
354. Mountjoy, M.G., Migraine mitigated by manipulation. *Clin. Trends Osteopath. Med.,* 4:1–3, 1977.
355. Vernon, H., Vertebrogenic migraine. *J. Can. Chiropract. Assoc.,* 29:20–24, 1985.
356. Vernon, H., Chiropractic manipulative therapy in the treatment of headaches: a retrospective and prospective study. *J. Manipulative Physiol. Ther.,* 5:109–112, 1982.

Index

C

F

G

H

I

J

K

L

M

R

S